Fundamentals of Diagnostic Imaging

Fundamentals of Diagnostic Imaging

An Introduction for Nurses and Allied Health Care Professionals

Edited by Anne-Marie Dixon

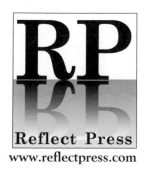

Reflect Press
www.reflectpress.com

First published in 2008

ISBN: 978 1 906052 10 2

British Library Cataloguing in Publication Data
A catalogue record for this book is available from the British Library

The authors and publisher have made every attempt to ensure the content of this book is up to date and accurate. However, health care knowledge and information is changing all the time so the reader is advised to double-check any information in this text on drug usage, treatment procedures, the use of equipment, etc. to confirm that it complies with the latest safety recommendations, standards of practice and legislation, as well as local Trust policies and procedures. Students are advised to check with their tutor and/or mentor before carrying out the procedures in this textbook.

Production project management by Deer Park Productions

Typeset by PDQ Typesetting

Cover design by Oxmed

Printed and bound by Cromwell Press Ltd, Trowbridge, Wiltshire

Distributed by BEBC, Albion Close, Parkstone, Poole, Dorset BH12 3LL

Published by Reflect Press Ltd
11 Attwyll Avenue
Exeter
Devon, EX2 5HN
UK
01392 204400

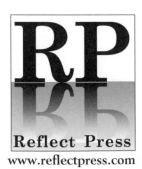

www.reflectpress.com

Contents

Author Biographies

Jamie Beck

Jamie Beck is currently a lecturer at the University of Bradford. After graduating as a radiographer in 2000, Jamie spent five years in clinical practice at Airedale General Hospital, West Yorkshire before moving into education. He completed a postgraduate certificate in Higher Education Practice in 2007. Jamie teaches on a wide range of subjects within the undergraduate radiography programme and contributes to the University's inter-professional learning strategy – a subject on which he has presented at both national and international conferences. Jamie's particular areas of special interest include e-learning, radiography education and forensic radiography – he has had several articles published in *Synergy*, the monthly magazine of the Society of Radiographers and is a member of the Association of Forensic Radiographers.

Elaine Chaplin

Elaine Chaplin graduated as a radiographer from the University of Bradford in 1998. She has worked in clinical practice in several hospitals in the West Yorkshire region as well as spending a year working in New Zealand. Since 2005 Elaine has been a lecturer in radiography at the University of Bradford, teaching on the undergraduate radiography programme with involvement in the delivery of interprofessional education.

Elaine's professional background is in angiography and she developed and leads a postgraduate certificate and diploma programme in vascular imaging and intervention at the University of Bradford. Elaine is a member of the Yorkshire and Trent regional committee of the Society of Radiographers.

Stephen Boynes

Stephen Boynes is an experienced radiographer and teacher with over 20 years academic experience. During the last 10 years he has been responsible for teaching magnetic resonance imaging (MRI) to undergraduate student radiographers and other health care professionals in the School of Health Studies at the University of Bradford. He is also currently the postgraduate course coordinator for the Division of Radiography and has particular responsibility for leading the team delivering the postgraduate certificate in magnetic resonance imaging pathway. Stephen has been the College of Radiographers' representative on the Consortium for the Accreditation of Clinical Magnetic Resonance Education and was the recipient of a mid-career professional development award from PPP Healthcare Medical Trust which used to further develop his knowledge and skills in MRI.

Gillian Clough

Gillian Clough qualified as a diagnostic radiographer in 1988. Following this she worked at Bradford Hospital Trust for three years before moving to the Leeds & Wakefield Breast Screening Service where she undertook further training in mammography. After another three years Gillian moved to St James's University Hospital Leeds and stayed there until 2003 setting up their dedicated Breast Imaging Department, developing Advanced Practice roles for mammographers working in symptomatic breast imaging and obtaining a Master in Breast Imaging award from the University of Leeds. Gillian was an associate lecturer at the University of Leeds from 1997 to 2003 where she helped to develop and deliver post-graduate courses in breast imaging; since 2003 Gillian has held a substantive post as university teacher at the University of Bradford where she contributes to teaching imaging science and technology on the undergraduate radiography programme and runs a post graduate module for stereotactic breast biopsy.

Anne-Marie Dixon

Anne-Marie Dixon moved into post as senior lecturer in breast imaging at the University of Leeds in April 2008 after spending six and a half years as lecturer/senior teacher in the Division of Radiography at the University of Bradford. Anne-Marie qualified as a radiographer in 1984 obtaining the Diploma of the College of Radiographers (CoR) and went on to further specialist clinical practice and study gaining the CoR Diploma in Medical Ultrasound in 1992. Subsequently she has obtained Master's degrees in both Medical Ultrasound and Research Methods for Social Sciences, and a postgraduate certificate in Higher Education Practice.

Anne-Marie's areas of specialist clinical practice include gynaecological and breast ultrasound; she is an established lecturer and publisher in these areas and still undertakes clinical practice sessions in local hospitals. Anne-Marie is an active member of the British Medical Ultrasound Society having served on their Scientific and Education committee and Publications committee, being Editor of the Society's peer reviewed journal *Ultrasound* from 2007- 2008. Anne-Marie is currently a member and vice-chair of the Society of Radiographers' Ultrasound Advisory Group.

Fiona Ware

Fiona Ware qualified as a diagnostic radiographer in 1978 at Leeds General Infirmary. She moved to St James's University Hospital, Leeds in 1981 and into their newly established Diagnostic Imaging Unit soon after to undertake computed tomography examinations. While there, Fiona discovered Nuclear Medicine. Fiona was awarded a formal qualification in Nuclear Medicine – the College of Radiographers' Diploma in Radionuclide Imaging – in 1983 and has since worked continuously in this discipline participating in a broad spectrum of clinical imaging, reporting and supervisory roles – she was departmental manager from 1986 to 1991 and is currently an Advanced Practitioner Radiographer in Nuclear Medicine in the St James's Institute of Oncology, Leeds. Since 1984 Fiona has been involved in work-based clinical tutoring and student supervision and has contributed to the teaching of nuclear medicine technology and imaging techniques on undergraduate radiography programmes in Leeds, Bradford and Sheffield. From 1999 – 2007 Fiona was formally seconded to the Bradford University Division of Radiography as a practitioner lecturer and then was employed as a University Teacher where, as course leader, lecturer and clinical supervisor, she ran the postgraduate Diploma in Nuclear Medicine. Fiona has a particular interest in Positron Emission Tomography. She has co-authored a number of published articles, poster presentations and proffered papers.

Andy Scally

Andy Scally qualified as a diagnostic radiographer in 1984 and worked in Ireland and Croydon before studying for a degree in Physics at Birkbeck College, University of London. Andy has worked in radiography education at the University of Bradford since 1992, in which time he has obtained Master's degrees in Physics and in Medical Statistics. His main areas of interest and expertise are in physics and technology of medical imaging, radiological protection and quantitative research methods in medical research. In collaboration with colleagues in the Medical Physics Department at Bradford Royal Infirmary, Andy was instrumental in developing the University of Bradford's Radiation Protection Supervisors' training course, to which he is a key contributor.

Gary Culpan

Gary Culpan qualified as a diagnostic radiographer from the Bradford School of Radiography in 1990 and, after working at Bradford Hospitals for a short while, spent 10 years at St James's University Hospital in Leeds. Gary was one of the first radiographers chosen to train to report Accident and Emergency (A&E) radiographs as part of a Department of Health-funded project which ran between 1992 and 1995 and subsequently undertook definitive reporting of A&E musculoskeletal radiographs. During that time he also trained to undertake barium enemas and, in 1997, he undertook a research role and became course leader for the Leeds barium enema course for radiographers. In 1998 Gary was a co-founder of the gastrointestinal radiographers' special interest group (GIRSIG) and remains an active participant. He joined the teaching team at the University of Bradford in December 2001 and alongside undergraduate teaching in image interpretation runs post graduate courses in musculoskeletal, chest and abdomen and gastrointestinal image reporting. Gary still undertakes regular clinical sessions performing and reporting barium enemas and is a key trainer for the University's newly installed CR and PACS system.

Jane F. Williams-Butt

Jane Williams-Butt initially trained as a therapy radiographer in Glasgow in 1974, then re-trained as a diagnostic radiographer and subsequently worked for nine years in the Western Infirmary, Glasgow. After a career break, she moved to Leeds and worked in several posts before joining the pioneering computed tomography (CT) team at St James's University Hospital, helping to establish their exemplary CT unit. From Leeds, Jane moved to Bradford Hospitals as the superintendent radiographer in the CT department and oversaw development of the service from a one-unit installation to a multi-unit suite. Fourteen years later Ninewells Hospital in Dundee lured her back to Scotland with an offer to be Radiography Manager, her current position.

Jane is an honorary lecturer on the Bradford University CT course and is a former examiner for the Dublin CT course. She is known nationally as a lecturer on head CT reporting courses such as those provided by the University of Central England and Dundee University. One of Jane's other main specialist interests is CT colonography. From 2005-2008 Jane served as a Health Professions Council partner.

Terry Lodge

After qualifying as a diagnostic radiographer Terry Lodge developed special interests in theatre and mobile radiography and later trained in computed tomography. Terry spent four years as a hospital-based clinical tutor during which one of his priorities was to develop student skills in caring for patients undergoing diagnostic imaging examinations. Terry subsequently became a full-time lecturer at the Bradford School of Radiography, which was later incorporated into Bradford and Airedale College of Health. In 1995 Terry moved with the Division of Radiography to the University of Bradford. After joining the University Terry held the post of clinical education co-ordinator for undergraduate students working closely with clinical staff to develop effective systems for student supervision and assessment of clinical skills competence. Terry took particular interest in developing students' reflective learning abilities to enable them to self-assess their ability to care for all patients equitably. As a senior lecturer in the division Terry eventually took on the role of course leader for the BSc (Hons) Diagnostic Radiography programme.

Terry is involved in interprofessional education initiatives and has an interest in collaboration with health and social care disciplines. Throughout his career as a radiographer and lecturer he has taught pre-registration nurses about radiography and the care of patients undergoing imaging examinations – a topic he believes to be an essential element of high quality seamless care and interprofessional collaboration in provision of services.

Acknowledgements

All photographic images of 'patients' and health care staff have been simulated; the authors would like to thank the following colleagues for participating in this: Elaine Chaplin, Gillian Clough, Gary Culpan, Anne-Marie Dixon, Helen Harcus, Mandy Lyons, Salma Parveen, Danuta Spence, Aisling Spencer, Pam Thompson, Sarah Turner, Fiona Ware and Alan Wormald.

Introduction

This book has been written by a team of experienced radiographers and university lecturers with responsibilities for delivering undergraduate BSc (Hons) Diagnostic Radiography programmes and a wide range of post-graduate courses in specialist medical imaging techniques such as computed tomography, magnetic resonance, nuclear medicine, radiographic image interpretation and medical ultrasound. The team also has experience of introducing the principles of diagnostic imaging across a wide range of other nursing, allied health care and medical education and training programmes, and it is from this experience that this book has arisen.

Although much of the material in the book is available elsewhere, students would typically need to access small introductory sections of a wide range of large and expensive specialised texts in order to find it. Unable to find a suitable single text to recommend to their students, the authors have devised their own in-house teaching materials and these form the basis of the content of the book.

Starting with Chapter 1 – General radiography, the reader is taken through the full range of radiation based diagnostic imaging investigations that are commonly encountered in a hospital imaging department, such as fluoroscopy – Chapter 2, computed tomography – Chapter 3 and radio-nuclide imaging – Chapter 4. Additional chapters cover non-radiation based techniques such as ultrasound – Chapter 5 and magnetic resonance imaging – Chapter 6.

In general, each of the chapters first provides a simple and accessible description of the underlying physical principles of the imaging technique and explains how the equipment works. In the second half of the chapter, the authors describe the most common clinical conditions investigated with the technique using 'case studies' of fictitious patients to illustrate typical clinical signs and symptoms and the most commonly diagnosed abnormalities and pathologies.

With radiation based imaging presenting a potential hazard to both patients, accompanying persons and health care staff, Chapter 7 outlines the biological basis of such hazard and reassures the reader by explaining how risk is minimised and balanced against the potential benefit for the patient.

As NHS services are modernised and patient care pathways are stream-lined, it is no longer only medical doctors who request imaging investigations and receive the results – Chapter 8 explains the processes involved in appropriately referring patients for imaging tests and explains what information a health care worker can expect to find in an imaging investigation report.

Chapter 9, although last in the book is not the least important. It is here that imaging investigations are considered from the patient's point of view, looking at issues such as consent to investigation and the use of chaperones. In this chapter patients, and those helping them prepare for investigations and recover from image-based interventional procedures, will find explanatory information about why they might need to starve or drink copious amounts of fluids or water beforehand.

In all the chapters, explanatory diagrams and photographs have been used alongside simulated patient scenarios and real life clinical images, to illustrate the written text. Throughout the book, technical 'jargon' has been kept to a minimum while still introducing readers to commonly used specialist terminology. Interested readers are directed to appropriate further reading at the end of each chapter.

It is hoped that this book will be readily accessible and affordable and that it will appeal to a wide range of people intending to be, or currently training to be, health care workers; this might include those studying GCSE Advanced level sciences, those enrolled on GNVQ / Foundation degrees in health and social care, and nursing and allied health professions' Foundation and BSc degrees and Diploma courses such as, for example, radiography and physiotherapy. The relatively simple style of the book might also give it appeal to members of the general public who want to know a little bit more about their own imaging investigations.

Chapter 1

General Radiography
Gillian R. Clough and Jamie Beck

INTRODUCTION

In 1895 Wilhelm Conrad Roentgen discovered **X-rays** and produced the world's first ever radiographic image of a human being, reputed to show his wife's hand (Olson, 2002). The medical profession was quick to see the potential for this new technology and it has featured prominently in patient care ever since. Although there have been technical advances over the years that have improved image quality and reduced radiation hazards to staff and patients, the basic principles of general radiography have not changed.

WHAT ARE X-RAYS?

X-rays are one of seven types of electromagnetic radiation that make up the electromagnetic spectrum (see Table 1.1). Although different in the way they behave, all seven types of radiation have some common characteristic features (see Box 1.1). The wavelength of radiation in the electromagnetic spectrum decreases from the longest – radio waves – through to very short wavelength gamma rays; as wavelength decreases the energy of the radiation increases. Some of the higher energy radiations, X- and gamma rays and some ultraviolet light, cause ionisation and are collectively referred to as **ionising radiation**. Ionising radiation is a potential biological hazard because, for example, some cancers are caused by exposure to ionising radiation – so work involving use of these radiations is governed by legislation. In the United Kingdom (UK) the Ionising Radiations Regulations (1999) (IRR) and the Ionising Radiation (Medical Exposure) Regulations (2000) **(IR(ME)R)** cover this.

Case study

Richard was a bit worried about having a radiograph of his hand because he had heard that X-rays were dangerous. He asked Olivia, the radiographer, if it was really necessary and if it could give him cancer. Olivia explained that although large doses of radiation are dangerous, small amounts of radiation can be very useful– in Richard's case it would help the doctors make an accurate diagnosis and help them choose the right treatment. She explained that when the doctor decided to request the radiograph of Richard's hand they had thought very carefully about it and decided that the risk of him getting cancer was very small and that the risks to Richard from not knowing what was wrong with his hand or giving him the wrong treatment were greater.

Technical note

In the United Kingdom approximately 135,000 people die from cancer every year. If everyone in the UK (population 60.6 million, 2006) had a radiograph of their hand, an extra 30 people might die of cancer later on in life as a result. The radiation dose received by any individual during radiography of the hand is very small and is equivalent to what they would normally receive over 1.5 days from natural back-ground radiation (radioactive materials in the ground, in food and from outer space!). People are 40 times more likely to die from being knocked down by a car, and 100 times more likely to die as a driver or passenger in a car, than they are to die from cancer as a result of having a hand radiograph.

(MHRA 2007, Moir 2005, HPA 2001, ONS 2005, 2007)

Radiation risks and benefits are discussed in detail in Chapter 7.

How are X-rays produced?

Some X-rays occur naturally and travel to Earth from the sun or even from beyond our solar system. The process of **radioactive decay** also sometimes results in the emission of X-rays. In medical radiography, X-ray **photons** are produced in a controlled manner through the rapid deceleration of fast-moving electrons in an **X-ray tube**.

An X-ray tube contains a **cathode** at one end, separated by a short distance from an **anode** at the other end – these are encased in an evacuated glass tube (see Figure 1.1). To produce X-rays, a current is supplied to the cathode and a high potential difference, in the kilovoltage (kV) range, is applied between the anode and the cathode. Free electrons, which have a negative charge, are released by the cathode and are strongly attracted to the positively charged anode. As they accelerate across the vacuum they gain a considerable amount of kinetic energy before crashing into the

Name	Wavelength (m)	Examples of production	Some uses
Radiowaves	$10^{-1} - 10^6$	Oscillating electrons in an aerial	Radio transmission
Microwaves	$10^{-3} - 10^{-1}$	Electron tube oscillators Lasers	Radar Microwave cooker TV transmission
Infrared radiation	$7 \times 10^{-7} - 10^{-3}$	Natural and artificial heat sources	Heat detectors Night vision camera TV remote control
Visible light	$4 \times 10^{-7} - 7 \times 10^{-7}$	Natural and artificial light sources	Vision Photography
Ultraviolet light	$10^{-8} - 4 \times 10^{-7}$	The sun	Sunbed Viewing security marker
X-rays	$10^{-13} - 10^{-8}$	Bombarding metal with electrons	Security scanner Diagnostic and therapeutic radiography
Gamma rays	$10^{-16} - 10^{-10}$	Radioactive decay	Food preservation Equipment sterilisation Radiotherapy

Table 1.1 The electromagnetic spectrum (Graham and Cloke, 2003, Thomson and Wakeling, 2003)

- Have transverse wave form
- Carry energy
- Can travel in a vacuum
- Have a constant speed of 3×10^8 ms^{-1}
- Are unaffected by electric and magnetic fields
- Travel in straight lines
- Obey the inverse square law
- Have frequency, wavelength and amplitude

Box 1.1. **Common characteristics of electromagnetic waves** (Dowsett *et al* 2006)

anode. The anode contains an inlaid **target** area, usually made of tungsten, and when the electrons strike this their kinetic energy is converted into heat and X-radiation. If the electrons interact with the nuclei of the tungsten atoms a **continuous spectrum** of X-ray photon energies is produced. If they interact with the orbiting electrons of the tungsten atoms, **line spectra** of discrete photon energies are produced (see Figure 1.2). X-ray production is an inefficient process – only 1 per cent of the initial tube energy is converted into X-ray photons (Dendy and Heaton, 1999), with most of the energy converted into heat, which is absorbed by

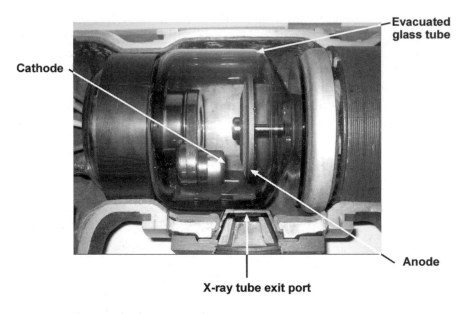

Figure 1.1 Photograph of an X-ray tube insert

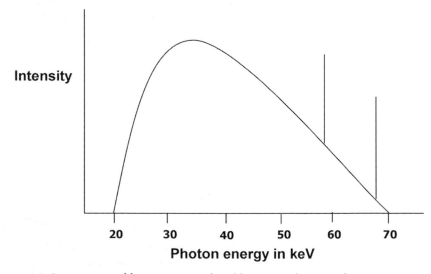

Figure 1.2 Continuous and line spectra produced by a general X-ray tube operating at 70keV

the anode. Typical **X-ray exposures** in medical imaging occur over fractions of a second – this is the time for which a patient might be asked to keep still or hold their breath. To prevent small areas of the target overheating the anode usually rotates at high speed during X-ray production – the noise of this can be heard by patients when the **radiographer** pushes the button to start the exposure.

The target area is built into the edge of the anode and is aligned obliquely so that most of the X-rays produced are directed out through a small area of the X-ray tube's glass cover towards the aperture or **exit port**. However, since X-rays are emitted in all directions from the target, the rest of the glass tube has to be surrounded by a lead lined metal case – the X-ray tube housing. The X-ray tube housing is manipulated by the radiographer to direct the X-ray beam that emerges through the exit port towards the patient.

Case study

When Richard was having his hand X-rayed after he had fallen playing football, he asked Olivia, the radiographer, why she was shining the light from the X-ray tube onto his hand. Olivia explained that this was a **light beam diaphragm** and that it helped her see and control the position and area of the X-ray beam. Olivia explained that the visible light source was aligned with the X-ray beam so she could see the location of the X-ray beam on the surface of a patient's body. She continued to tell him that by opening and closing a lead-lined shutter, making the light (and the X-ray beam) area larger or smaller, she could make sure that all of his hand would show up on the image and that the area of his body irradiated was kept as small as possible.

What happens as X-rays pass through the body?

As the X-ray beam passes through a patient's body, some X-ray photons are completely absorbed (i.e. all their energy is transferred to the body), some are scattered (they transfer some of their energy to the body and emerge with less energy and in a different direction) and some pass straight through the body unaltered (see Figure 1.3).

In diagnostic radiography the term **attenuation** is used to describe a transfer of energy from the X-ray beam into the body; this occurs due to **photoelectric absorption** and **Compton scattering**. Both these processes involve X-ray photons interacting with the orbital electrons of atoms in the patient's body.

Photoelectric absorption is proportional to the third power of the atomic number (atomic number cubed) of the attenuating material and is inversely proportional to the third power of the X-ray photon energy (see Equation 1.1).

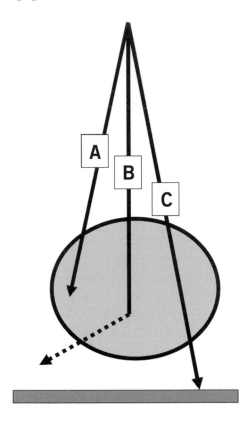

Figure 1.3 Possible outcomes when X-ray photons interact with body tissues. A: total absorption – no X-ray energy emerges from patient; B: scattered (secondary) radiation – X-ray photon emerges from patient with reduced energy and in a random direction; C: primary radiation – X-ray photon passes through patient unaltered in energy and direction

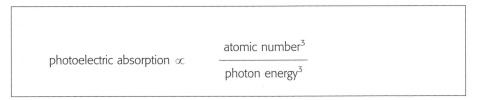

$$\text{photoelectric absorption} \propto \frac{\text{atomic number}^3}{\text{photon energy}^3}$$

Equation 1.1 Photoelectric absorption (from Farr and Allisy-Roberts, 1998)

It is this effect that is predominantly responsible for producing the characteristic 'shadow pattern' that represents bodily structures in the X-ray image. The human body consists of a wide range of tissue types, each of which has a specific average atomic number depending on the constituent elements of the cells in the different tissues. Fat and muscle tissue, with relatively low average atomic numbers (6 and 7.4 respectively (Farr and Allisy-Roberts, 1998)), typically exhibit little photoelectric absorption – X-ray photons easily pass through unaltered, compared with bone with an average atomic number of 13 (ibid). When imaging soft tissue specifically, very low X-ray photon energies are used to maximise the effect of photo-electric absorption.

Compton scattering is essentially independent of the atomic number of body tissue but is inversely proportional to X-ray photon energy (see Equation 1.2).

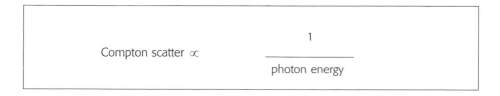

$$\text{Compton scatter} \propto \frac{1}{\text{photon energy}}$$

Equation 1.2 Compton scattering (from Farr and Allisy-Roberts, 1998)

As the direction of scattered radiation is fairly random in relation to the position of bodily structures it affects the image indiscriminately and thus, because it does not contribute to an accurate representation of anatomical structure, scatter degrades the diagnostic quality of radiographic images. The radiographer therefore has to think about the thickness of tissue the X-ray beam needs to pass through and the average atomic number and density of the tissues being demonstrated when they choose the **exposure factors** for each examination.

Radiographic exposure factors are chosen so that sufficient X-ray photons pass through the patient and form an image on a **detector** placed behind or beneath the patient. The average photon energy of the X-ray beam must be controlled to give good **differential absorption** in tissues – this will produce an image with **radiographic contrast** so that different organs and bodily structures are visualised at different **radiographic density** levels. **Contrast agents** are sometimes introduced into the body to alter the natural/inherent attenuating properties of tissues – these techniques are discussed in detail in Chapter 2.

Case study

When she was X-raying Richard's hand, Olivia used two halves of one detector plate to get views of the bones in two different positions. After asking Richard to put his hand in the first position on one half of the detector, she carefully adjusted the light beam diaphragm to make sure the X-ray beam only irradiated his hand and one half of the detector. She placed a piece of lead rubber over the other half of the detector during the exposure to 'mask' the area not being used.

Technical note

Radiographers try to reduce the amount of scattered radiation produced by limiting the X-ray beam so that it only irradiates the area of interest. They also use lead rubber to absorb scattered radiation and stop it reaching the detector and affecting the image.

How is the radiographic image captured, viewed and stored?

Having passed through the patient's body, the X-ray beam has been modified – it contains image information as variations in photon intensity over its cross-sectional area (see Figure 1.4). The variations in energy are captured by an image detector and are converted into a suitable format for storage and display (viewing).

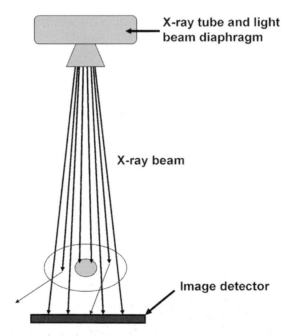

X-ray tube and light beam diaphragm

X-ray beam

Image detector

Figure 1.4 X-ray transmission through a patient onto an image detector

Traditionally, radiographic images have been captured using direct exposure radiographic (photographic) film or using radiographic film with **intensifying screens.** Similar to conventional photography, the film has to be kept in a light tight box (in radiography this is known as the **cassette**), and then the film has to be processed before viewing. Direct exposure film has a very high **spatial resolution** – it produces very detailed images but, unfortunately, it requires high radiation doses to achieve adequate film blackening. As a consequence its clinical use in modern radiography practice is restricted to some dental examinations and to **dosimetry** (monitoring the radiation dose to health care workers).

Intensifying screens – thin sheets of plastic coated on one side with a luminescent compound – can be attached to the insides of the film-holding cassette. Intensifying screens emit light when irradiated and enhance the blackening effect of X-ray photons – this allows adequate film blackening with much less radiation and therefore at much lower radiation doses to the patient. Until the mid-1990s film/screen radiography was the most commonly used image detection system for general radiography.

When using radiographic film systems however, only one copy of the image is produced. This might get lost and, once acquired and processed, the image cannot be manipulated or adjusted in any way. Acquiring images in a digital format overcomes these limitations. Digital radiographic imaging systems have been available for several years and are now being introduced across the UK as part of the government's *Connecting for Health* programme (DoH, 2005).

Computed radiography (CR) systems are similar to conventional radiographic imaging systems in that they use a plate coated with a luminescent compound – the **photostimulable image plate,** in a cassette (see Figure 1.5), although there is no need for radiographic film. The luminescent

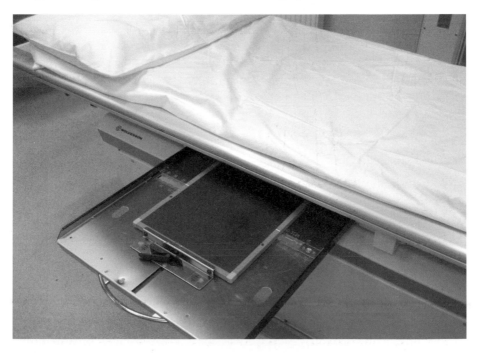

Figure 1.5 A CR cassette placed in an X-ray couch cassette tray

compound used in photostimulable plates (barium fluorohalide) absorbs X-ray photons during the radiographic exposure. Although some energy is emitted immediately as light photons, most of the X-ray energy is absorbed and stored on the CR plate. The cassette is then taken to a 'reading' device that removes the CR plate and scans it with a laser. The stored energy is then released as light photons – a process known as photostimulable emission – and the emitted light is channelled to a **photomultiplier tube**. The varying light signal is then converted into a varying electronic signal by the photomultiplier tube, and is digitised and stored as digital data.

As with conventional film/screen systems, the CR cassette with its photostimulable plate has to be changed between exposures. **Digital radiography** (DR) systems use a fabricated electronic array that remains in situ between exposures and thus makes image acquisition quicker and more efficient.

The fabricated electronic array or **digital detector** is an integral component of the radiographic equipment. The system either converts X-ray energy into light (using something similar to intensifying screens) and then into electrical charge (using **photodiodes**) – an **indirect digital** system – or converts X-ray photon energy directly into electrical charge – a **direct digital** system. Both systems store the variable electrical energy profile on a matrix of small capacitors.

The image information, in the form of differential charges stored in the capacitor array, is read out a **pixel** (capacitor) at a time, again giving a varying electrical signal that is digitised and stored. The system is 'cleared' electronically; i.e. the capacitors are discharged after each examination, ready for the next exposure without having to physically change a cassette.

Digital image capture and storage has many advantages over conventional photographic film-based radiography. In particular, once a digital image has been acquired it can be manipulated electronically – the image can be made lighter or darker, its contrast (**grey-scale** range) increased or decreased, and parts of the image can be magnified or cropped. This allows images to be optimised for each particular examination and can prevent the need for further exposures and additional patient irradiation.

How is the radiographic image viewed?

Radiographic images can be viewed as **hard copy** images or **soft copy** images. A hard copy image is an image or images on a sheet of film. These may have been acquired using a traditional film/screen system or may have been printed from a stored digital image. Hard copy images should be placed on a traditional X-ray viewing box and viewed with transmitted light (see Figure 1.6).

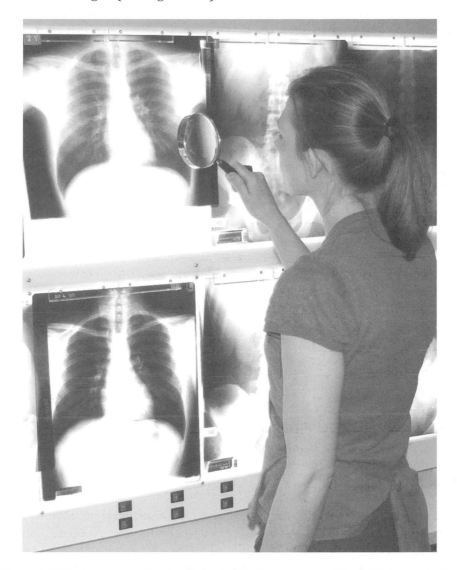

Figure 1.6 Viewing a conventional radiographic film image on a traditional X-ray viewing box

Soft copy images are viewed on a television (TV) monitor. The monitor may use either cathode ray tube (CRT) or flat panel liquid crystal display (LCD) technology. Although CRT technology traditionally had better spatial resolution, dedicated high quality flat panel LCD monitors can now be made that are of adequate quality for viewing and reporting diagnostic images (see Chapter 7).

With the widespread installation of digital imaging systems, the 'filmless' hospital is becoming more common. Sophisticated computer systems – Picture Archiving and Communications Systems (**PACS**) – now store, manage and distribute image files and there is no longer the need for vast libraries of medical images on conventional radiographic film. With appropriate networking, PACS can interface medical imaging with other hospital information systems, can centralise the storage of all imaging files within a hospital, and sometimes across multiple sites within a hospital Trust, and can allow multiple users to view the same image at various locations at the same time. PACS allow images to be stored and transmitted between hospitals and indeed across the globe, thus facilitating the concept of **telemedicine**.

How are patients prepared and positioned for radiographic examinations?

Patients require minimal preparation for general radiography – they will often be asked to take off their own clothes and wear a plain thin hospital examination gown. This is important as it prevents any **artefacts**, such as buttons, zips, keys or money in pockets, appearing on the image and obscuring the view of body structures. Although examination gowns are available whenever needed to maintain a patient's dignity, occasionally creases and seams will produce artefacts so radiographers will often try to avoid covering the area under examination if this is possible – typically the lower arms, lower legs and a man's chest will be examined without any covering.

Due to the geometry of X-ray beam production there is always some magnification and geometric unsharpness (blurring) in the radiographic image (see Figure 1.7). To keep this to a minimum patients are usually positioned with the structures under investigation as close as possible to

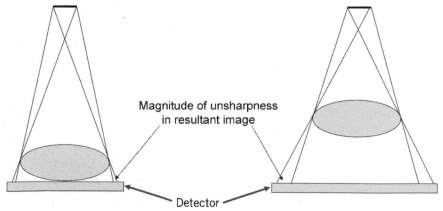

Figure 1.7 Magnification and geometric unsharpness – as the distance between an object and the detector increases, the object appears more magnified and more blurred in the image

the image detector. This gives better spatial resolution and allows more accurate measurements to be made. When a large area of the body is being imaged, for instance an adult's chest, or the body part is a long way from the image detector, for instance when the side of the neck cannot be positioned close to the detector because of the shoulders, the X-ray tube is positioned quite a long way from the patient to help reduce magnification and geometric unsharpness (see Figure 1.8).

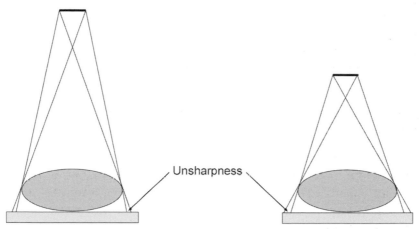

Figure 1.8 X-ray tube position and geometric unsharpness – increasing the distance between the X-ray tube and the object reduces magnification and geometric unsharpness

Case study

When Deborah was having her abdomen X-rayed, Olivia the radiographer took great care to position her to give the best view of the body parts under investigation, in this case her kidneys and bladder. Once she had done this Olivia asked Deborah to keep very still and explained that if she moved before the radiograph was exposed it might mean that she was in the wrong position and it may not be possible to make an accurate assessment and reach a diagnosis. Just before she made the exposure, Olivia asked Deborah to hold her breath and reminded her to keep very still. Once Olivia had heard the noise which indicated the exposure was over, she told Deborah to breathe again and relax.

Technical note

Just as in conventional photography moving subjects result in blurred images, so movement during the exposure will produce a blurred radiograph and might result in the exposure having to be made again. When the lungs or abdomen are being X-rayed patients are asked to hold their breath to reduce the likelihood that the images will be blurred by organs moving during respiration.

What are the clinical uses of general radiography?

In comparison with many other diagnostic imaging tests, general radiography is relatively quick, economical and accessible and is relatively straightforward for the patient. Despite the radiation dose incurred it is often used as a first-line investigation, following clinical evaluation, to eliminate sinister pathology or serious trauma and, as such, sometimes allows doctors to offer patients a safe **conservative treatment** plan. For many patients general radiography is the only imaging investigation required and quickly gives reassurance that all is well. General radiography can be used to evaluate both bone and soft tissue structures and allows the diagnosis of a wide range of conditions; it will also identify those patients who require more complex, more expensive, or higher radiation dose imaging investigations in order to reach a diagnosis.

General practitioners readily refer patients for radiography to help them diagnose and manage disease, children and athletes often require radiography following accidents or sporting injuries and it is unusual for anyone to be admitted to hospital without having at least one radiograph along the way. The challenge faced by many X-ray departments is ensuring that radiography is only used when it can realistically be expected to have an important effect on patient management and, as such, that its use does not contribute to population radiation dose unnecessarily. The **Royal College of Radiologists** regularly issues up-to-date evidence-based guidelines to help clinicians decide which imaging investigation is likely to be most appropriate for any particular patient (RCR, 2007).

The most common radiographic examinations are of the chest and limbs. These have a relatively low radiation dose and are the examinations of choice in the first instance when lung disease or bone injury is suspected. General radiography will not readily demonstrate the soft tissue structures of the central nervous system (i.e. the brain or the lymphatic) blood vessels and organs of the digestive and urinary systems), without the use of contrast agents (see Chapter 2). Radiography is essentially a technique for diagnosing structural, i.e. anatomical, abnormalities, although the long-term effects of abnormal physiology, i.e. function, degenerative and metabolic diseases, can sometimes be seen.

Chest radiography

The most commonly performed radiographic examination is the chest X-ray – over eight million people a year in the UK have a chest X-ray (Watson *et al.*, 2005). The chest radiograph gives a general overview of the soft tissues of the heart and lungs and the surrounding bony thoracic (rib) cage (see Figure 1.9a). It is ideally performed with the patient stand-

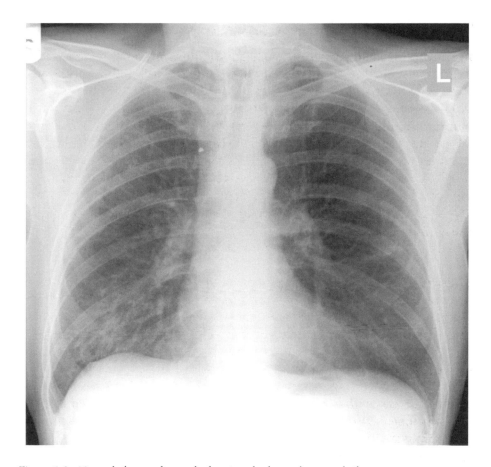

Figure 1.9a Normal chest radiograph showing the heart, lungs and rib cage

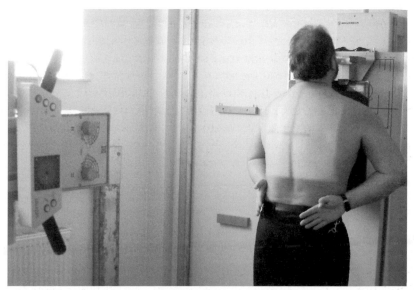

Figure 1.9b The patient is positioned facing the cassette for a PA (postero-anterior) chest X-ray

ing facing the image detector (see Figure 1.9b) so the heart is not magnified too much, and after expanding the lungs. A deep breath in, fills the lungs with air and ensures the air-filled spaces are seen in good radiographic contrast to blood vessels which are filled with fluid.

If this can be achieved the heart size (cardio-thoracic ratio – CTR) and shape can be assessed and the lungs checked. Any lung areas that are not filled with air such as, for example, where there is a solid tumour, where the lung has collapsed, or contains fluid or infection, should be spotted easily. Chest X-rays are used to diagnose diseases such as **pneumonia**, tuberculosis and heart failure, to monitor degenerative diseases such as **chronic obstructive pulmonary disease (COPD)**, and to see how well patients are responding to treatment. They are also used for **screening** patients prior to surgery if they are at high risk of anaesthetic complications.

Orthopaedic (bone) radiography

Radiographs of bones are used to demonstrate fractures, dislocations, tumours and **degenerative diseases** such as arthritis. Since a single radiographic projection produces a two-dimensional image of a three-dimensional object, radiographs are usually taken in two planes to show the bones and the alignment of joints and fractures (see Figure 1.10). Typically two images are obtained at right angles: one from the front – an **antero-posterior (AP) projection** – or one from the back – a **postero-anterior (PA) projection** – and one from the side – a **lateral projection** (see Figure 1.11). This helps to give the doctors an idea of the three-dimensional nature of any problem and helps them plan how to manage and treat injuries. Serial or check radiographs are used to verify the position and healing of fractures following manipulation (pulling back into alignment), fixation (inserting orthopaedic screws or nails) and/or immobilisation (application of a plaster cast). Radiography is also commonly used to check the position of artificial joints immediately after they have been inserted and to check them later on if loosening or infection is suspected.

Occasionally pain and discomfort are caused by bone tumours – although a **biopsy** (tissue sample) is required to be absolutely sure of the type of tumour, radiographic appearances (density and outline) can indicate the most likely diagnosis.

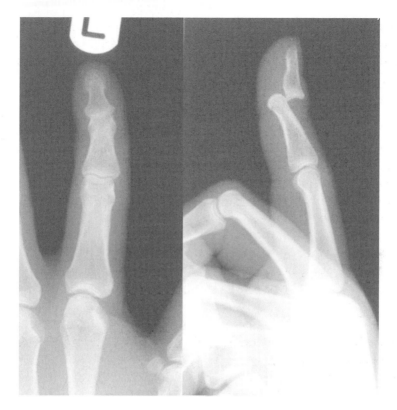

Figure 1.10 Postero-anterior (PA) and lateral projections of an index finger: two projections at right angles are required to fully appreciate the dislocation

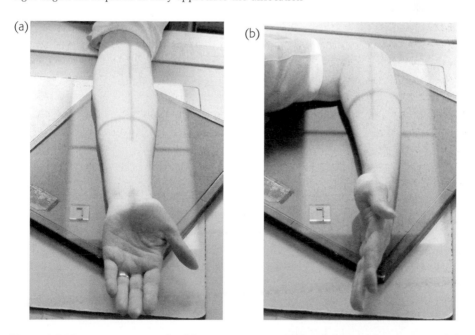

Figure 1.11 Patient positioning for (a) antero-posterior (AP) and (b) lateral projections of the forearm

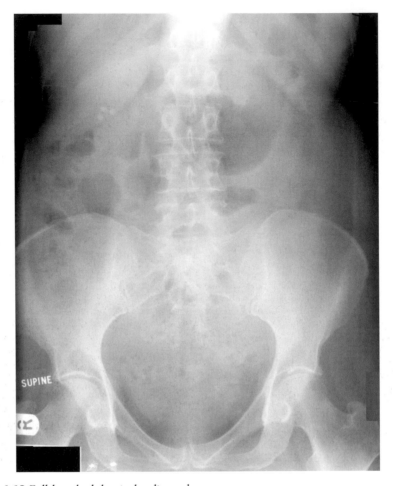

Figure 1.12 Full length abdominal radiograph

Abdominal radiography

In the past, the abdominal X-ray was a useful initial test when doctors suspected patients had **gallstones** or **kidney stones**. A relatively large area of the abdomen can be demonstrated on one radiograph (see Figure 1.12) – this usually includes the lower ribs, spine and pelvic bones as well as most of the soft tissue of the lower digestive and urinary systems, i.e. the large and small bowel, and the kidneys, ureters and bladder (KUB).

While the abdominal radiograph will show a large proportion of gall-stones and kidney stones, **computed tomography** (see Chapter 3) and **ultrasound** (see Chapter 5) are now considered to be more sensitive tests, with ultrasound having the advantage of not involving ionising radiation. However, when patients present with severe abdominal pain, suggestive of bowel obstruction or perforation, the plain abdomen radiograph is still the most appropriate first-line test.

Dental radiography

Quite a lot of people will have had an X-ray performed by their dentist. Specialist 'orthopantomogram' equipment, which circles around the patient's head, is used to image the upper and lower jaws and all the teeth at once (see Figure 1.13). To image individual teeth, small plastic-covered dental radiography film or a small digital detector is placed inside the patient's mouth. Dental radiography will demonstrate tooth decay, impacted wisdom teeth, retained roots and jaw fractures. Other specialised orthodontic radiographs are used by maxillo-facial surgeons to assess and monitor upper and lower jaw alignment.

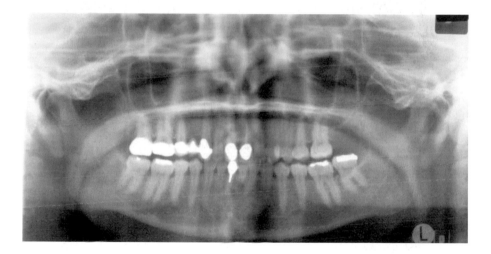

Figure 1.13 An orthopantomogram showing the upper and lower jaws and all the teeth

Foreign bodies

General radiography can be used to locate foreign material that has been inserted (pushed), inhaled (breathed), or ingested (swallowed) into the body and is sometimes used to facilitate the accurate positioning of **catheters** and other tubes and drains (Figure 1.14).

Whether or not foreign material can be seen depends on its density and atomic number in comparison to that of the body part in which it lies. Objects such as metallic bullet fragments and carpentry nails will be obvious, while plastic or wooden foreign bodies, such as children's toy parts, may not readily show up. Some medical catheters have a thin filament or coating at the tip to help them show up. Computed and digital radiography allows image manipulation to increase the chances

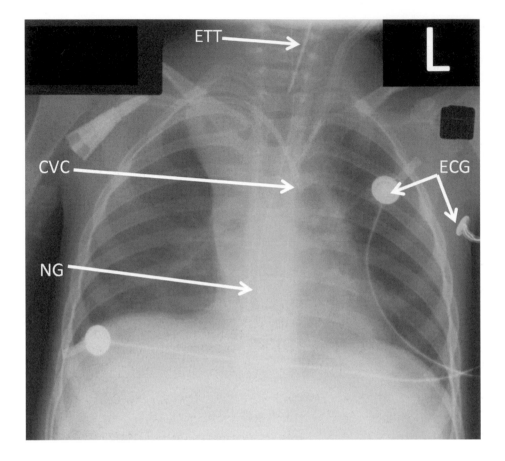

Figure 1.14 A chest radiograph from an unconscious patient in the intensive care unit showing the position of the breathing tube (ETT: endotracheal tube), the feeding tube (NG: nasogastric tube) and monitoring lines (CVC: central venous catheter, ECG: electrocardiograph leads)

of demonstrating foreign bodies and any associated soft tissue (ligament, muscle, blood vessel) damage.

Increasingly, particularly in areas near air or sea ports, radiography is used to identify 'bodypacking' – the practice of ingesting or inserting illegal drugs or precious stones into the body in inert packaging.

SUMMARY
The use of general radiography is limited by the hazards associated with exposure to ionising radiation, poor **contrast resolution** for soft tissue and its two-dimensional nature, which leads to the superimposition of overlying structures. Soft tissue structures are better demonstrated using contrast agents (see Chapter 2). Superimposition can be reduced by angling the X-ray tube or using a variety of patient positions. Cross-sectional imaging techniques such as computed tomography (see Chapter 3), ultrasound (see Chapter 5) and magnetic resonance imaging

(see Chapter 6) potentially give better contrast resolution and three-dimensional spatial awareness. MRI and ultrasound do not expose patients to ionising radiation.

The potential benefits of any diagnostic imaging examination must outweigh its associated risks. With good radiographic technique and appropriate imaging protocols, the radiation dose for general radiography can be kept minimal (RCR, 2007). The technique is accessible and cost-effective and continues to be useful in the diagnosis and management of many diseases and trauma.

FURTHER READING

Allisy-Roberts, P.J. and Williams, J. (2008) *Farr's Physics for Medical Imaging* (2nd Ed). Philadelphia: Saunders Elsevier
This book covers the physics of X-ray production and interaction as well as radiation protection issues, and explains the modes of operation of all the main imaging equipment.

Dowsett, D.J., Kenny, P.A. and Johnston, R.E. (2006) *The Physics of Diagnostic Imaging* (2nd Ed). London: Hodder Arnold
Provides very good in-depth explanations of how imaging equipment works.

Graham, D.T. and Cloke, P. (2003) *Principles of Radiological Physics* (3rd Ed). London: Elsevier Churchill Livingstone
This gives good explanations of X-ray production and interaction and covers radiation protection issues. It also includes text on the basic physics required for a full understanding of X-ray production and interaction.

Gunn, C. (2002) *Bones and Joints: A Guide for Students* (4th Ed). Edinburgh: Churchill Livingstone
A good guide to radiography of the skeletal system (bones) with anatomical diagrams and labelled radiographic images.

Sutherland, R. and Thomson, C. (2007) *Pocketbook of Radiographic Positioning* (3rd Ed). London: Churchill Livingstone
A useful guide to standard radiographic positioning and technique. Contains anatomical photographs with corresponding radiographic images.

Chapter 2

Fluoroscopy, Contrast Agents and Image-guided Intervention
Elaine Chaplin and Gary Culpan

INTRODUCTION

General radiography is used to obtain single 'snapshot' images of the body when it is stationary – static images. **Fluoroscopy** is a radiographic (X-ray based) technique used to image the body, or a structure within the body, when it is moving – dynamic imaging. Fluoroscopy allows body movement to be watched as it is happening, namely in 'real-time'. Static images may be recorded at various times during a dynamic examination, by asking the patient to keep still and hold their breath just like in general radiography, but moving images can also be recorded as 'video clips'. In addition to evaluating anatomical structure, dynamic imaging allows some observation of bodily function.

Although dynamic images viewed on TV monitors are still two-dimensional, movement of the fluoroscopic equipment and/or the patient during the examination shows anatomical structures and relationships between structures from different perspectives, giving the viewer more of an awareness of the three-dimensional nature of the body.

In this chapter we will initially describe how fluoroscopy equipment differs from that used for general radiography and then go on to give examples of some clinical applications of the technique. Since many dynamic anatomical systems in the body consist of soft tissue structures that are not normally seen well on radiographs, we also include a comprehensive review of radiographic **contrast agents** in this chapter.

FLUOROSCOPY EQUIPMENT

A fluoroscopy unit is comprised of an X-ray tube connected and centred to either an **image intensifier** (established technology) or a digital detector (recent development), a processing unit and a closed circuit TV monitor (see Figure 2.1).

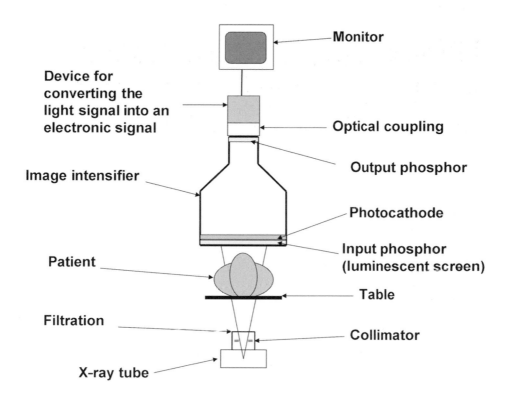

Figure 2.1 Diagram of an image intensifier based fluoroscopy unit

In general radiography, X-rays are produced for only a fraction of a second during an **exposure**, whereas in fluoroscopy X-rays are produced over a much longer period of time. The radiation dose to the patient is minimised by using a very low X-ray tube current that produces a low intensity X-ray beam.

When the X-ray beam emerges from the patient's body it hits the image intensifier and is absorbed by a layer of luminescent material which then emits light. This light is absorbed by a photocathode, which then emits electrons. The electrons are accelerated towards, and focussed onto, a much smaller area of luminescent material. When the electrons strike this it emits light. This second image is smaller and much brighter than the first – hence the name image intensifier. The intensified light image is converted to a varying electronic signal and used to generate an image for viewing on a TV monitor. Dynamic and static images are recorded digitally on the fluoroscopy system itself and can then be archived onto digital optical or compact discs. Hard copy static images may be printed onto sheets of film and dynamic images may be viewed as soft copy movie clips on a TV monitor.

Radiation protection for staff

Health care staff performing and assisting during fluoroscopy often have to stay close to the patient, who is a source of **scattered radiation**, during the examination so they wear protective clothing such as aprons and thyroid shields that have lead rubber in them. The lead (atomic number 82) attenuates radiation and reduces the radiation dose to staff – typically lead rubber devices offer protection equivalent to a 0.25-0.35 mm thickness of lead. Although radiation intensity is very low during fluoroscopy, it is much higher during the acquisition of permanent static or dynamic images. Staff who must remain close to the patient during these exposures will also wear protective goggles and may stand behind small mobile screens containing lead equivalent material when this happens. Adherence to local radiation protection rules and appropriate use of protective clothing and equipment ensure the staff radiation dose is kept as low as reasonably achievable and is not hazardous to their health.

CONTRAST AGENTS

Fluoroscopy is occasionally used to look at how body structures move during respiration (breathing) or to see what happens when a joint, such as the knee or shoulder, moves. More often it is used to look at the anatomical structures that move blood, food and urine through the body. Since most anatomical structures making up these 'dynamic' systems are soft tissue and are surrounded by other tissues or organs of similar radiographic density, fluoroscopy is usually combined with the use of contrast agents – substances introduced into the body to alter the natural **radiographic contrast**.

Contrast agents introduced into blood vessels (arteries or veins) show how blood travels through the cardio-vascular (heart and blood vessel) system – a technique known as **angiography**. Contrast agents introduced into the gastrointestinal (digestive) tract show how food moves down the oesophagus (food pipe), into the stomach and through the small and large bowel (intestines and colon). Some contrast agents are filtered by the kidneys and eliminated from the body in urine. While this is happening the kidneys, ureters and bladder are visible on conventional radiographs; this is the basis of the intravenous urogram or IVU examination (see Figure 2.2).

Principles of contrast agent use

In 'general' radiography, it is difficult to distinguish separate soft tissue structures when there are a number of such structures lying closely together. For example, the liver, gall bladder and right kidney all lie in

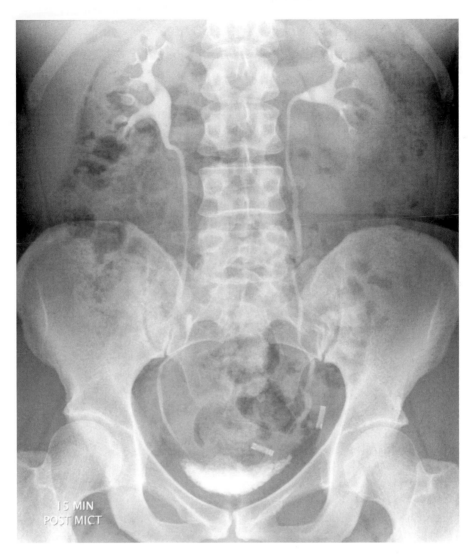

Figure 2.2 During an intravenous urogram (IVU) examination the right and left kidneys, ureters and bladder are visible on conventional radiographs following the intravenous administration of water-soluble iodine based contrast agents

the right upper quadrant of the abdomen and appear as similar density on radiographs. They are thus not easily seen as separate structures and this makes conventional radiography of limited value in detecting structural abnormalities of soft tissue. Some organs of the body contain cavities, for example the heart chambers and urinary bladder, or channels, for example the blood vessels and gastrointestinal (GI) tract. If these are filled with a simple biological fluid such as blood or urine, or are collapsed and empty, they will not show up on conventional radiographs – this then makes it difficult to tell if there is any abnormality inside the organs or any malfunction in the normal filling, emptying or transit time.

To make soft tissue structures and bodily cavities or channels more 'visible', i.e. to make them 'stand out', contrast agents are introduced into the blood passing through the organs or into the cavity or channel. Contrast agents can be used to increase the density compared with surrounding structures or to reduce the density to less than that of surrounding structures. A 'positive' contrast agent has a high atomic number and attenuates more X-rays than the surrounding anatomical structures. A 'negative' contrast agent has a lower atomic number than the surrounding anatomy and thus allows more X-rays to pass through.

Types of contrast agent

Contrast agents can be naturally occurring agents or pharmaceutical products. Gas (air) trapped in the stomach and bowel acts as a naturally occurring negative contrast agent and helps demonstrate the stomach cavity and bowel lumen in good radiographic contrast to the rest of the abdominal contents (see Figure 2.3). Often, as people get older, calcium (atomic number 20) begins to build up in their blood vessels. This acts as a natural positive contrast agent and is particularly useful for showing when the major blood vessel in the abdomen – the aorta – is enlarged by an **aneurysm** (see Figure 2.4).

Most fluoroscopy examinations use positive pharmaceutical contrast agents either alone or in combination with negative ones like, for example, the **double contrast** barium enema (see below). Positive pharmaceutical contrast agents have some general and some particular characteristics that make them suitable for specific fluoroscopic examinations (see Box 2.1).

Diagnostic properties
- Concentrates in the required anatomical area.
- Appropriate consistency to fill or flow through the body system of interest.
- Easily and quickly eliminated from the body after the examination.

Practical characteristics
- Easy to administer to the patient.
- Not too unpleasant for the patient.
- Relatively inexpensive.
- Readily available.
- Safe:
  - no long-term side effects;
  - not poisonous;
  - a stable preparation that does not break down within the body.

Box 2.1 Desirable properties of a contrast agent

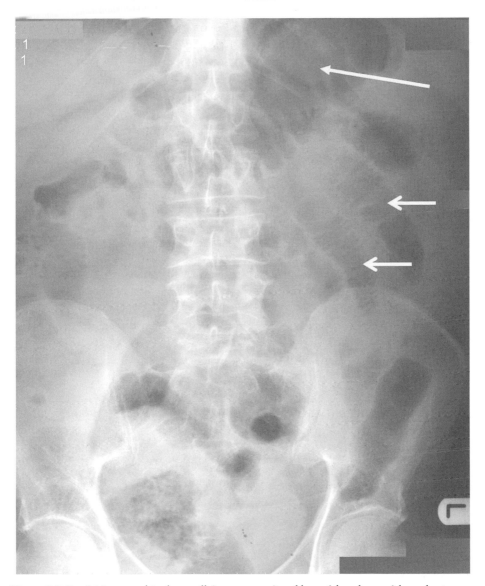

Figure 2.3 Gas (air) trapped in the small (open arrows) and large (closed arrow) bowel acts as a naturally occurring negative contrast agent and helps demonstrate the bowel lumen in good radiographic contrast to the rest of the abdominal contents

Choice, administration and elimination of contrast agents

A wide range of pharmaceutical contrast agents is used in diagnostic medical imaging. For each patient and each examination the **radiologist** will choose the one that is most suitable for the organ or system of interest and the routes available for introducing it into the body (see Table 2.1). The amount and concentration of contrast agent used will also depend on an individual patient's weight, the relative size of the organ of interest and the route used to administer the preparation.

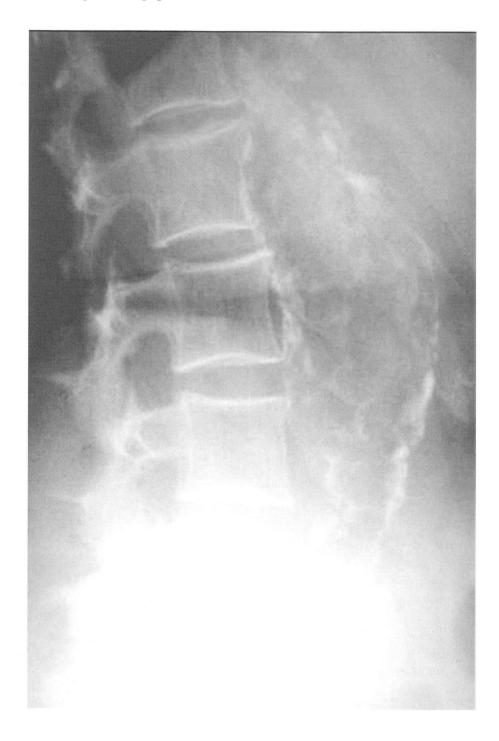

Figure 2.4 Calcium in the walls of blood vessels acts as a natural positive contrast agent and outlines an abdominal aortic aneurysm (widening)

Target organ/ system	Pharmaceutical preparation/ natural contrast	Example of product trade name	Concentration: density (weight/ vol per cent or iodine concen- tration (mg ml^{-1})	Negative or positive	Route of administration into body
Arteries	water-soluble iodine based	Ultravist/ Omnipaque	300–370	Positive	Injection intra-arterial intravenous
Arteries (below diaphragm)	CO_2			Negative	Injection intra-arterial
Brain (computed tomography – CT)	water-soluble iodine based	Ultravist	300	Positive	Intravenous injection
Bile ducts	water-soluble iodine based	Ultravist	150	Positive	Via needle or tube directly into the bile ducts
Large bowel – colon (barium enema)	barium sulphate suspension	E-Z HD	100 per cent w/v	Positive	Enema – into rectum
Double contrast examination	Air/ CO_2	Not applicable		Negative	Enema – into rectum
If perforation (leak) is suspected	water-soluble iodine based	Urografin/ Ultravist	150	Positive	Enema – into rectum
Oesophagus (barium swallow)	barium sulphate suspension	E-Z HD	250 per cent w/v	Positive	By mouth
If perforation (leak) is suspected	water-soluble iodine based	Ultravist/ Omnipaque	150-300	Positive	By mouth
Gynaecology – female reproductive	water soluble iodine based				Directly into uterine cavity
Angiography/ embolisation	water-soluble iodine based	Ultravist/ Omnipaque	300	Positive	Intra-arterial/ intravenous injection
Small bowel – intestines (small bowel meal)	barium sulphate suspension	E-Z Paque	60-100 per cent	Positive	By mouth
Small bowel enema	methylcellulose			Negative	Directly into the small bowel via a nasojejunal (intestinal) tube
Stomach (barium meal)	barium sulphate suspension	E-Z HD	250 per cent w/v	Positive	By mouth
	CO_2	Carbex granules		Negative	By mouth
Urinary – kidneys, ureters and bladder (IVU examination)	water-soluble iodine based	Ultravist/ Omnipaque	350–370	Positive	Intravenous injection
Cystogram (bladder only)			150–300	Positive	Directly into cavity of bladder using a catheter
Veins of the leg or arm (venography)	water-soluble iodine based	Ultravist/ Omnipaque	150–300	Positive	Intravenous injection

Table 2.1 Types of contrast agents used in radiological procedures

Pharmaceutical contrast agents may be introduced directly into a body cavity and some can be injected into blood vessels. For the GI tract, fluid suspensions of barium (atomic number 56) sulphate are usually given by mouth (as a 'swallow' or as a 'meal'), or are instilled into the rectum as an 'enema'. Water-soluble iodine (atomic number 53) based contrast agents are usually administered into the blood stream as either an intra-arterial or intravenous injection (rapid administration) or as an infusion (slow administration). Water-soluble iodine based contrast agents can also be administered through a **sinus** (abnormal opening into the body) or **fistula** (abnormal connection between two channels in the body).

Water-soluble iodine based contrast agents that have been administered into the blood stream are filtered out by the kidneys and excreted from the body in the urine. Barium sulphate suspension is biologically inert so it is not absorbed through the bowel wall – the contrast agent remains in the GI tract and is eliminated during the natural excretion process.

Contrast agent side effects

Although radiographic contrast agents have been rigorously tested just like all other commercially available pharmaceutical products (medicines), occasionally they do have side effects. Serious reactions to barium sulphate are rare – the most common side effect of this contrast agent is constipation. Patients will be encouraged to drink plenty of fluid after barium examinations to help eliminate the contrast agent and prevent impaction – they will also be warned that the barium sulphate is white and will colour their faeces for a few days. Barium sulphate suspension cannot be used in the GI tract if the patient has recently had gastrointestinal surgery or if the doctor suspects there might be a **perforation**, or hole, in the GI tract wall. This is because barium sulphate suspension is not absorbed by the body and thus any that leaks into the abdominal or chest cavity cannot be eliminated. Any barium sulphate suspension that escapes from the GI tract will cause pain and shock, and occasionally a patient may die if this happens.

As water-soluble iodine based contrast agents injected into the blood stream are excreted via the kidneys it is important to check a patient's kidney function before administering them. Approximately 5 per cent of patients will suffer kidney damage from a contrast agent examination – this is more likely in patients who are dehydrated, have **multiple myeloma** or **diabetes mellitus**, and those given very large doses of contrast agent, but patients known to have poor renal function already are at highest risk (Chapman and Nakielny, 2001, p.33). Of particular note, patients taking the drug Metformin® (usually for diabetes) will be asked to stop taking it for 48 hours after a water-soluble contrast agent examination and their renal function (**creatinine** levels) will be closely monitored. Metformin® and water-soluble iodine based contrast agents are both excreted by the kidneys and in combination can 'overload' kidney function with fatal consequences.

Some patients are sensitive to iodine and may have an allergic reaction. Allergic reactions vary in severity (see Table 2.2) and occur most commonly with an intra-arterial or intravenous injection of water-soluble iodine based contrast agents.

Magnitude of reaction	Effect on patient
Mild	Hot flush Metallic taste in mouth Nausea (feeling of sickness) Sneezing
Moderate	Erythema (development of raised red skin patches) Urticaria (development of itchy skin lumps) Vomiting
Severe	Anaphylactic shock – severe allergic reaction which may lead to: • heart irregularity or heart attack (cardiac arrest); • swelling and constriction of the respiratory tract; • bronchospasm and cessation of breathing (respiratory arrest).

Table 2.2 Side effects of water-soluble iodinated contrast agents

Reactions usually occur very quickly after administration of the contrast agent, although some delayed reactions (up to two days later) have been observed. The development of iodine-based contrast agents over the years has reduced the incidence of serious reactions. Incidence of mild reactions is now about one in every 30 patients and moderate reactions occur in approximately one in 100 patients (Kessel and Robertson, 2005, p.13). Patients who have reacted previously, those with known allergies (particularly to shellfish) and those with hyper-sensitivity conditions such as asthma and hay fever, should be considered at higher risk of a more serious reaction. Water-soluble iodine based contrast agent mortality is approximately one in 40,000 patients (Kessel and Robertson, 2005, p.13).

Before giving a contrast agent to a patient the radiographer and **radiologist** will ask the patient a series of questions and/or check their notes to help identify if they are at increased risk of reaction and to make sure that the examination is absolutely essential. Prophylactic (preventative) drugs such as antihistamines and steroids are sometimes given to reduce the risk of an allergic reaction in high risk patients. In some cases alternative imaging techniques, such as ultrasound or magnetic resonance imaging, can be used and sometimes alternative contrast agents (for example, carbon dioxide) can be substituted.

Case study

Tony, a 64-year-old male, was referred to the imaging department as an out-patient to have a femoral (thigh) angiogram to assess **peripheral vascular disease** in his legs. When Dr Stephens, the radiologist, asked about allergies Tony told him that he had a bad allergic reaction to an iodine based water soluble contrast agent when he had an IVU four years before.

Dr Stephens explained that it was possible to do the examination using alternative contrast agents this time. First of all he said he could go ahead there and then and use carbon dioxide (CO_2) – a negative contrast agent. He then explained that this would show the blood vessels in Tony's legs almost as well as the standard iodine based contrast agent. As an alternative, Dr Stephens also suggested that Tony could come back on another day and have the test done with magnetic resonance imaging – a magnetic resonance angiogram (MRA) using a different type of contrast agent called gadolinium (see Chapter 6). Tony said he had already arranged his work commitments around having the test done that day so he preferred to go ahead immediately and asked Dr Stephens to use the CO_2.

Technical note

Carbon dioxide dissolves in the blood and is eliminated from the body during normal respiration. However, it cannot be used for intra-arterial injections to examine structures above the diaphragm as it can interfere with brain function (Kessel and Robertson, 2005, p.15).

In all radiology departments wherever and whenever contrast agents are being used emergency drugs and resuscitation equipment (a 'crash' trolley) are available. All radiographers are trained in basic life support and some are trained to administer emergency drugs: all are aware of what immediate action to take and how to summon help when a serious contrast reaction occurs.

CLINICAL APPLICATIONS OF FLUOROSCOPY

The barium enema

This examination is used to assess the 'large bowel' or colon. Typical pathologies demonstrated include diverticular disease (see Figure 2.5), polyps (see Figure 2.6) and colon cancer (see Figure 2.7).

During this examination, a semi-rigid **catheter** is placed in the patient's rectum and approximately 200 ml of liquid barium sulphate suspension is introduced. The patient is asked to turn from lying on their left side onto their front and then around onto their back so that the contrast agent can 'paint' the walls of the large bowel. Most of the barium sulphate is then drained out and the bowel is inflated, usually with a small manual air pump, so that the **lumen** (channel) expands and the inner walls can be seen clearly. The colon is visualised in 'real time' on the fluoroscopy monitor and several radiographic images are recorded during this, and sometimes afterwards, to demonstrate the entire large bowel including all its various 'twists and turns' (see Figure 2.8).

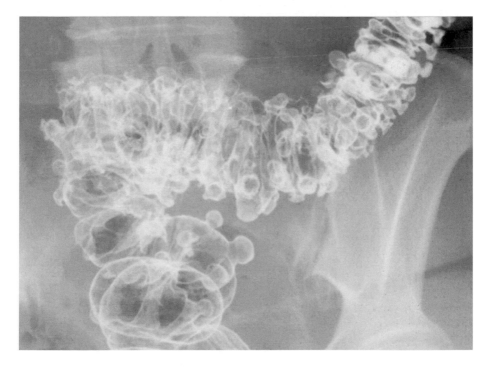

Figure 2.5 Diverticular disease (out-pouching of the bowel wall) as demonstrated during a double contrast barium enema examination

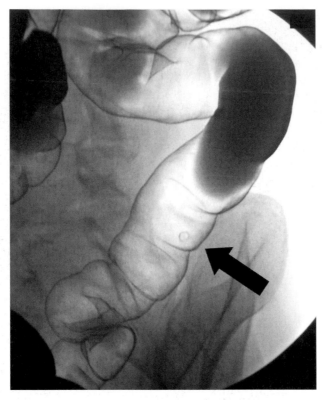

Figure 2.6 Pre-cancerous bowel polyps (arrow) can be demonstrated during a barium enema examination

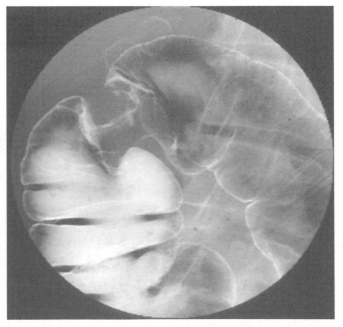

Figure 2.7 Barium enema examination demonstrating colon cancer – the 'apple-core' appearance in upper left quadrant of image

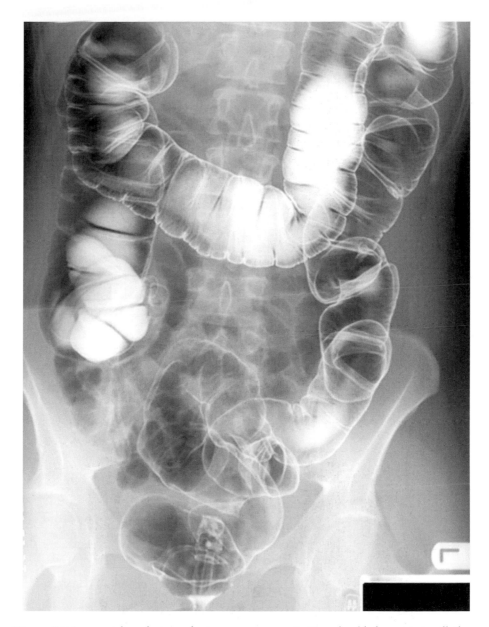

Figure 2.8 Images taken during a barium enema examination should demonstrate all the 'twists and turns' of the colon

Case study

Margaret, a 62-year-old lady, visited her doctor because her bowel habit had recently changed and she was now having constipation for several days followed by diarrhoea. She also told her GP that she occasionally got some pain and a bloated feeling in her lower abdomen.

Margaret's GP suspected that something was causing a partial blockage in her bowel so he sent her for abdominal radiography. When the report came back it said that nothing abnormal had shown up but that the soft tissues of the bowel are not clearly seen this way. The report suggested that Margaret be referred for a double contrast barium enema if the GP was still suspicious that there might be some pathological cause for her symptoms.

A few days later Margaret received her barium enema appointment letter. She was surprised when she read the preparation instructions – it seemed rather complicated for what the GP had described as an 'X-ray test'. Margaret had to follow a special 'no residue' diet for two days before the test and one day before the test had to take some laxatives that had been sent from the hospital. When she arrived at the hospital for her appointment Sheila, the radiographer, asked lots of questions about Margaret's general health and also asked whether the laxatives had worked. Margaret said they had been very strong – she had not dared to stray out of her flat! Sheila reassured Margaret that this was a good result as it was very important that the bowel was completely clean before the examination.

At the beginning of the examination Sheila asked Margaret to lie on her left side on the examination couch so that a small tube could be inserted into her rectum. This was connected to a longer tube attached to a bag of barium sulphate liquid. When Sheila had checked that Margaret was ready for the test to start, the barium sulphate liquid was allowed to flow down the tube and into Margaret's colon. At first she felt a bit strange but that feeling soon wore off and Margaret assured Sheila she was reasonably comfortable. Occasionally Sheila asked Margaret to roll into a different position on the couch while part of the fluoroscopy machine was moved over her and Sheila watched the image on the TV monitor next to the couch.

A few minutes later, Sheila stopped the flow of barium sulphate and gave Margaret a small injection into a vein in her arm. Sheila explained that this would help relax the bowel and help prevent cramp-like pains for the next part of the examination. Following the injection, Margaret felt as if her abdomen was becoming 'blown up with wind' as Sheila gently pumped air through the rectal tube. Although it was a bit uncomfortable now, Sheila explained that Margaret should try not to let the air out until she had finished taking the images. Over the next five minutes Sheila asked Margaret to turn around and then keep still in various positions and to hold her breath occasionally while she looked all around the bowel and recorded various images.

Eventually Sheila informed Margaret that the examination was over and she could go to the toilet. Before she went home, Margaret was given a cup of tea and a biscuit and told that this would help her bowel start working normally again. The nurse gave Margaret a leaflet of instructions and pointed out where it said she should drink quite a lot over the next couple of days to 'flush the barium out' and remember to flush the toilet twice to prevent the barium sulphate causing a blockage.

A few days later the GP's receptionist telephoned Margaret and asked her to come in for her results. Margaret was relieved when the GP reassured her that the symptoms were not serious – the barium enema had shown that Margaret had some little pouches called 'diverticula' in her bowel. He explained that these would not be a major problem if she could increase the amount of fibre in her diet to help prevent them getting worse.

Interventional radiography

As well as diagnosing abnormalities, medical imaging techniques are also sometimes used to help treat disease conditions. Fluoroscopy allows needles, tubes and **catheters** to be introduced into the body while the radiologist and radiographer watch where they are going in the patient on the TV monitor. Fluoroscopic guided intervention can be used to:

- drain cavities – for example, cyst or abscess drainage;
- decompress blocked channels – for example, bile ducts in obstructive jaundice;
- widen narrowed channels – for example, arterial stenosis (angioplasty), bile duct stenosis (stent placement);
- place artificial devices – for example, heart pacemaker wires (see Table 2.3).

Where therapeutic procedures can be undertaken under image guidance this is often safer and quicker for the patient, and is more economical and less invasive that the alternative, which is often a traditional surgical operation. In addition, image-guided interventional procedures are usually undertaken as out-patient day case procedures in the radiology department (only occasionally is an overnight stay required); they usually only require local anaesthetic and thus have quicker recovery times.

Organ/ system	Procedure	Definition
Biliary (bile ducts)	Percutaneous transhepatic cholangiography/ drainage	Needle inserted through skin into liver to identify site of bile duct blockage and/or allow drainage
	Biliary stent placement	Positioning of a synthetic semi-rigid plastic or metal mesh tube to keep the main bile duct patent (open)
Cardiac (heart)	Insertion of pacemaker	Pacemaker wires threaded from shoulder veins into heart chambers and embedded into heart muscle to keep it beating regularly
	Cardiac angioplasty	Widening of narrowed (stenosed) coronary arteries – those supplying the heart muscle – by inflating and deflating a small balloon
	Cardiac stent placement	Positioning of a synthetic semi-rigid metal mesh tube in the coronary arteries to keep them patent (open)
Gastro-intestinal (digestive)	Enteric stent insertion, e.g. oesophagus, colon	Positioning of a synthetic semi-rigid metal mesh tube in the lumen to keep it patent (open)
	Percutaneous endoscopic gastrostomy	Tube inserted through skin into stomach for feeding – position checked with **endoscope**
Renal	Nephrostomy	Needle/tube inserted through skin into kidney to drain obstructed kidney
	Renal embolisation	Artificial blocking of blood supply to a kidney tumour
	Ureteric stent placement	Placement of synthetic semi-rigid plastic or expandable metal mesh tube into the lumen to keep it patent (open)
Vascular	Angioplasty	Widening of narrowed blood vessel lumen by inflating and deflating a small balloon
	Arterial stent placement	Positioning of a synthetic semi-rigid metal mesh tube in an artery lumen to keep it patent (open)
	Endovascular aortic repair/graft	Positioning of artificial patch/semi-rigid metal mesh to reinforce widened/weakened aorta (major blood vessel in abdomen)
	Embolisation	Artificial blocking (occlusion) of a blood vessel – usually to block off the blood supply to a tumour
	Direct intravascular thrombolyisis	Injection of solutions to dissolve blood clots and restore blood supply/flow
	Intravenous filter placement	Positioning of an artificial metal mesh 'sieve' to catch blood clots (usually from the legs) and stop them reaching the lungs

Table 2.3 Interventional radiology procedures

Specialised equipment used during interventional procedures, for example the intravascular stents, angioplasty balloons and the wires used to steer the devices into position (guidewires), must be **radio-opaque** (visible in the image) so their position can be watched in 'real time' as they are guided into place inside the patient (see Figure 2.9). As the target organs are soft tissue structures, a water-soluble iodine based contrast agent is injected down a catheter that has been threaded over the guidewire to demonstrate the anatomy before, during and after the procedure. In angioplasty this helps to confirm that the **artery** has been successfully widened (see Figure 2.10) or in **stent** insertion that the device has been successfully deployed (see Figure 2.11).

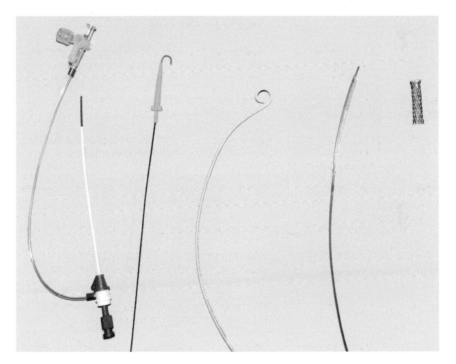

Figure 2.9 Examples of the specialised equipment introduced into blood vessels to widen narrowed arteries

Angioplasty (artery widening) and nephrostomy (kidney drainage) are two of the most commonly performed image-guided interventional procedures and can have a dramatic effect on the patients who receive them. They are performed under **aseptic conditions** in specially designed interventional fluoroscopy suites, similar to a day-case operating theatre, within the imaging department.

(a)

(b)

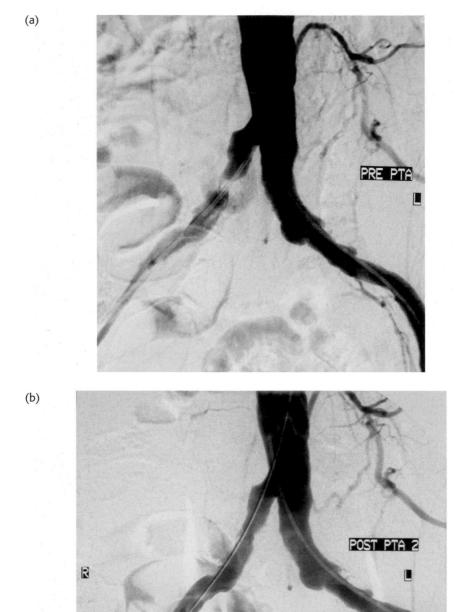

Figure 2.10 Fluoroscopy images taken during an angioplasty procedure confirm (a) that the balloon is positioned correctly at the stenosis (narrowed part), and (b) that the artery has been successfully widened

(a)

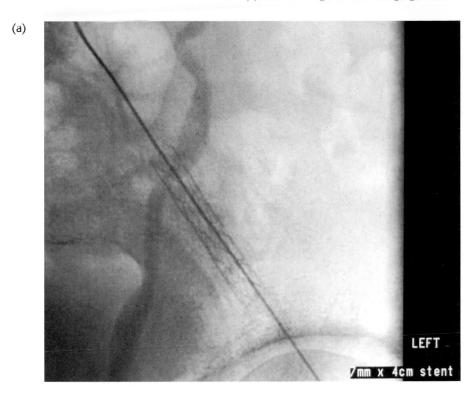

(b)

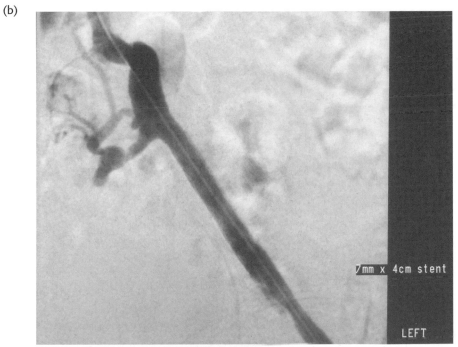

Figure 2.11 Fluoroscopy images taken during a stent insertion: (a) stent in position over guide wire, (b) contrast agent injection confirms successfully widened artery

Angioplasty

Angioplasty is an image-guided interventional procedure performed to widen the lumen of a blood vessel. The most common cause of **stenosis** (narrowing) is a build up of **atheroma** – fatty deposits and calcium on the inner walls of blood vessels. The procedure is called 'endovascular' as it is performed from inside the vessel as opposed to being performed from the outside as a traditional 'open' surgical procedure. The most common vessels treated are the coronary (heart) and the femoral (thigh) arteries – the procedure widens the artery and restores normal blood flow to the heart or legs respectively. Typically patients requiring angioplasty have symptoms of **ischaemia** (an inadequate blood supply). In the heart this manifests as **angina**, and in the legs the patient will suffer from **claudication**.

Most angioplasty procedures are performed using the femoral artery in the groin for access. This is a large superficial artery close to the abdominal aorta and allows guidewires and catheters to be passed through the arterial network to almost any diseased vessel (see Figure 2.12).

(a)

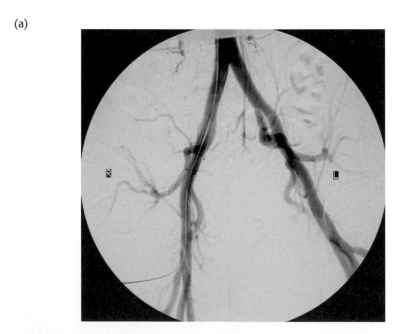

Figure 2.12(a) Most angioplasty procedures are performed using the femoral artery, a large superficial artery at the groin

After palpating the groin to identify the pulsating femoral artery, a large hollow needle is inserted through the skin until its end lies in the lumen of the vessel. A guidewire is then passed down the centre of the needle and advanced past the stenosed section of the artery. The needle is removed

(b)

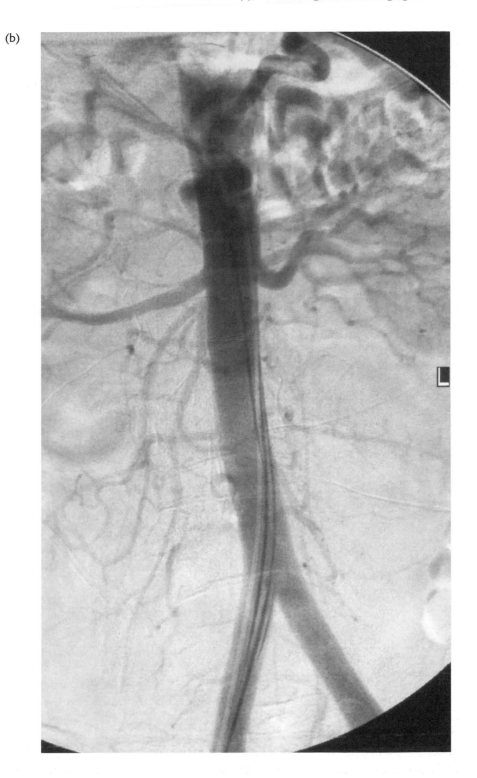

Figure 2.12(b) The femoral artery allows access via the iliac arteries to the aorta and its main branches

and a special angioplasty catheter is passed over the guidewire. The angioplasty catheter has a small balloon at one end; this is positioned exactly at the site of the stenosis and then inflated (using a contrast agent to make it visible on the image) so that it expands the narrowed vessel. Images are taken before and after the inflation to check how effective the procedure has been. Once the artery has been widened enough to restore good blood flow, the balloon is deflated and the catheter is removed. When the procedure is over, the radiologist presses their hand over the puncture site to compress the femoral artery against the bony pelvis until **haemostasis** (the cessation of bleeding) has been achieved.

Puncturing such a large artery is not without risk. The radiologist will check each individual patient's **clotting factors** before a procedure and will note their **international normalised ratio** (INR) value – this affects the size of puncture that can be safely made and the time that compression has to be applied to achieve haemostasis. It is not unusual for patients to have a haematoma (large bruise) after an angioplasty procedure but this invariably resolves naturally over time. More serious complications are rare and include:

- vessel rupture as the guidewire is placed or the balloon is inflated (this can happen if the balloon size has not been carefully matched to the vessel/stenosis diameter);
- the formation of blood clots (emboli) and thus blockages further down the vessel;
- the dislodging of atheroma and a subsequent embolic stroke – atheroma breaks off and travels down the arteries to block vessels supplying (parts of) the brain;
- pseudo-aneurysm formation – a false sac forms adjacent to the vessel as blood leaks out of the puncture site into the soft tissue space.

Case study

When Tony's wife came to pick him up a few hours after his angiogram, she discovered he had been lying flat in a bed in the Day Ward and she was pleased that he seemed to have recovered well. Once Suzy, the nurse, had checked that Tony's blood pressure and his temperature were normal, and that the small puncture wound at the top of his leg was not leaking through the dressing, Tony was allowed to go home. The nurse reminded Tony that he would get an appointment to see the doctor for the test results within the next few days.

Nephrostomy

Nephrostomy is performed when patients present with a kidney obstruction. Often a kidney stone (a renal or ureteric calculus) is blocking the normal flow of urine from the kidney down the ureteric tubes into the bladder. Urine volume builds up in the kidney and, if the blockage is not released, pressure builds up in the kidney, until eventually it will stop working and may be permanently damaged. During a nephrostomy, a 'pigtail' shaped catheter is inserted through the patient's back directly into the kidney collecting system – urine is then allowed to drain out via the catheter and is collected in a plastic bag attached to the end of the catheter.

Case study

Robert had been on the Admissions Ward for a week with severe low back pain and fever; his urine tests had shown high **creatinine** levels. When he had an IVU, Dr Stephens the radiologist told Robert that the cause of his symptoms had shown up – he had a stone (calculus) causing an obstruction of the left ureter.

Robert had been getting progressively worse for a couple of days when Mr Parker, the urologist (a doctor specialising in kidney disease), took him into the operating theatre to try to relieve the obstruction. Unfortunately this had proved unsuccessful as Mr Parker had been unable to get past the blockage by passing instruments up through Robert's bladder. Mr Parker explained to Robert that he had telephoned Dr Stephens in the imaging department and had asked him to put a tube into Robert's kidney through his back to drain the urine that was building up. Mr Parker explained that this should make Robert feel a lot better quite quickly and that it would also prevent his kidney becoming damaged any further. Gail, the Ward Sister, came to tell Robert that his procedure was booked for 3 p.m. that day and that he couldn't have anything to eat or drink after 11a.m. (four hours beforehand) to help prevent complications.

When Robert arrived in the imaging department, Dr Stephens asked him to lie on the fluoroscopy couch on his front with a pillow underneath him. Then Dr Stephens placed sterile drapes over Robert's back, cleaned the skin with an antiseptic solution and administered a local anaesthetic injection. Then, using both fluoroscopy and ultrasound (see Chapter 5) Dr Stephens guided a large hollow needle through Robert's skin and into the blocked kidney. He injected a small amount of iodine based water-soluble contrast agent to outline the collecting system of the kidney and to show how far down the ureter the stone was lodged.

Then Dr Stephens threaded a guidewire through the needle, removed the needle and threaded a catheter over the guidewire. Once the catheter was correctly positioned with its internal end in the collecting system, Dr Stephens secured it to Robert's skin with a small surgical stitch. Dr Stephens explained to Robert that this would ensure that it didn't come out. Finally, Dr Stephens put a sterile dressing over the wound and attached the external end of the catheter to a special plastic bag to collect the draining urine.

Robert was surprised when Dr Stephens told him the procedure was over – he hadn't really felt very much but over the next few hours he started to feel much better. Mr Parker was pleased that the nephrostomy had been possible because now he had more time to plan how he could sort out the blockage in Robert's ureter.

Technical note

Nephrostomy is usually only used as a temporary measure. Sometimes the obstruction will resolve spontaneously. Over a few days the stone may travel down the ureter and pass out through the bladder, and once urine is flowing naturally again, the patient can return to the imaging department to have the nephrostomy catheter removed.

Other image-guided interventional techniques

Image-guided intervention can be performed using ultrasound or computed tomography (CT) for guidance. Ultrasound (see Chapter 5) also gives 'real-time' visualisation and, because the equipment is relatively portable, is often used in conjunction with fluoroscopy to guide intervention. Ultrasound is particularly useful for locating solid organs such as the kidney during nephrostomy and the liver/bile ducts during percutaneous transhepatic cholangiography, or for obtaining solid organ **biopsy** samples. It is also useful for identifying those veins suitable for the insertion of **central venous catheters** that are used for intravenous feeding, drug administration and repeated blood sampling. Ultrasound is particularly attractive, where expertise exists, for image-guided intervention as it does not involve radiation.

When ultrasound visualisation is impaired, i.e. because of air in the lungs or the bowel, CT (see Chapter 3) can be used to guide **aspiration**, biopsy and drainage interventions. CT gives a more complete demonstration of cross-sectional anatomy and thus minimises the risk of inadvertent lung or bowel puncture.

SUMMARY

Fluoroscopy is an extension of the general radiographic technique that allows the visualisation of movement within the body. Combined with the use of contrast agents, fluoroscopy can be utilised to image a variety of soft tissue organs and structures – this is particularly useful for imaging the cardio-vascular, gastrointestinal and urinary systems of the body. Because fluoroscopy gives real-time visualisation it is used to guide a wide range of diagnostic and therapeutic techniques that involve the insertion of needles, wires and catheters into the body. Often image-guided interventional procedures can spare the patient a full-scale surgical operation and this means that diagnosis and treatment may be quicker, less painful and may not involve formal admission into hospital.

FURTHER READING

Chapman, S. and Nakieiny, R. (2001) *A Guide to Radiological Procedures* (4th Ed). Edinburgh: Saunders
This book explains in more detail how to carry out a wide range of common imaging procedures. It has a user-friendly format that clearly documents clinical indications, patient preparation, equipment and technique, aftercare and potential complications.

Dowsett, D.J., Kenny, P.A. and Johnston, R.E. (2006) *The Physics of Diagnostic Imaging* (2nd Ed). London: Hodder Arnold.
This book covers the principles and use of fluoroscopy units giving the reader an understanding of current systems and new developments.

Kessel, D. and Robertson, I. (2005) *Interventional Radiology – A Survival Guide* (2nd Ed). Edinburgh: Elsevier Churchill Livingstone
This gives a good overall introduction to interventional radiology techniques and procedures in the form of a step-by-step practical guide which also contains lots of diagrams and clinical photographs.

Chapter 3

Computed Tomography
Jane Williams-Butt

INTRODUCTION

Computed Tomographic (CT) scanning is a method of obtaining pictures (images) of anatomical cross–sections along the length of an area of the body. The scan is built up of individual 'slices' known as axial sections (the original name for the technique was 'CAT' scanning, standing for Computed Axial Tomography) lined up next to each other, a bit like the slices in a sliced loaf of bread. Although patients have been upset when radiographers make reference to taking 'slices' of them, there seems to be no other satisfactory expression and the term remains in common use in most imaging departments.

CT was invented by Sir Godfrey Hounsfield working with a team from Electric and Musical Instruments (EMI) and was first used in a clinical setting in 1972 at the Atkinson Morley Hospital in London. In 1979 he jointly received a Nobel Prize with Allan Cormack of Tufts University, Massachusetts, USA, who had been working independently on the same scientific principles.

THE TECHNOLOGY

A CT scanner (see Figure 3.1) has four major components: a table, the **gantry**, a computer and viewing/work stations. The scanning table has a rise-and-fall system that allows the patient to be lifted from chair height to the level of the centre of the gantry. The table top is also motorised so that the patient can be moved forwards or backwards a millimetre at a time or at speed. This allows the radiographer to position the patient very precisely according to the part of the body that is being imaged and according to the clinical question being asked, and it also allows the scanner to obtain several slices of information in a very short time.

The gantry is like a giant square doughnut and it contains all of the technical parts involved in acquiring the image. An X-ray tube within the gantry produces a thin beam of radiation that is absorbed to differing degrees depending on the type of tissue it travels through (see Chapter 1). A ring of **detectors** fixed around the periphery of the gantry picks up the radiation that has passed through the patient (see Figure 3.2). Complex electronic processing then converts the transmitted X-ray information into a CT image.

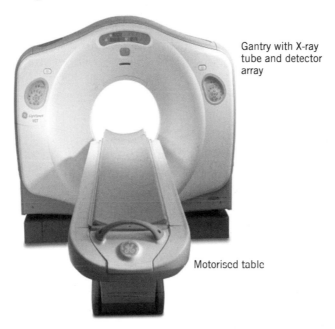

Gantry with X-ray tube and detector array

Motorised table

Figure 3.1 Modern-day CT scanner (image courtesy of GE Healthcare)

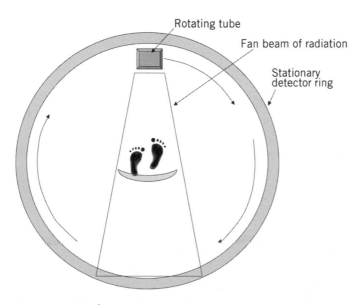

Rotating tube

Fan beam of radiation

Stationary detector ring

Figure 3.2 Diagram of a 4th generation CT scanning system with stationary detector array around the gantry

49

Computing power today is such that modern scanners can acquire 64 slices of information in 0.33 seconds. They can then store the data and can produce 20 images every second. Modern computer technology also allows images to be constructed in planes other than the plane of acquisition (see Figure 3). Thus, data acquired in the transverse (axial) plane can be processed to produce **coronal** and **sagittal** (lengthways) or oblique views. With the newest scanners, three-plane (multiplanar or 3-dimensional) reconstruction is routinely carried out in seconds. This **multiplanar reformatting** (MPR) gives additional diagnostic information without the radiographer having to rescan the patient in another position and without giving the patient any additional radiation dose. All the computer data and manipulation functions necessary to reformat images can be accessed at any viewing or work station.

Image data are stored as volume elements (**voxels**), the value of each being proportional to the amount of radiation that hits the detectors in the gantry after having passed through the patient. The data can be interrogated a voxel at a time to determine the amount of radiation absorbed by the corresponding anatomical volume in the patient's body – this **attenuation** is measured in **Hounsfield units** (HU). The computer assigns a different shade of grey to each HU value and these are used to produce a two-dimensional greyscale CT image to represent an anatomical cross-section of the body. The HU value, commonly known as the density, of any particular structure in the image helps the radiologist (a doctor specialising in imaging investigations) to determine the nature and type of the tissue it represents (see Figure 3.4). For example, if the CT computer cursor or mouse pointer is placed over an area in the image corresponding to bone, there will be a high HU reading (+240 for example). Air in the lungs usually has a value of minus 1000 HU, water density is 0, moving blood in vessels or in the heart has density of 40 but blood which has leaked out of vessels, i.e. that has haemorrhaged, is of higher density.

The HU value is a guide to how dense a fluid is and can help decide whether a patient needs additional imaging with **magnetic resonance imaging** (MRI) or a clinical therapeutic procedure. For example, if the HU value of an abscess is 0–15 HU it means it consists mainly of watery fluid and could be drained using a needle inserted through the skin. However, if the abscess contents are more dense, i.e. the HU value is higher than 25 HU, the fluid inside is thick and it may not be possible to drain it using conventional needles or **catheters** (hollow tubes inserted in to the body) – the patient may need an operation.

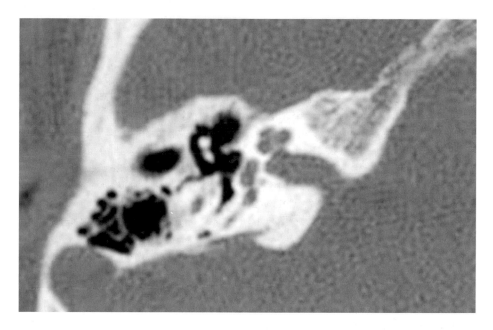

Figure 3.3a High resolution (0.6 mm slice thickness) axial plane CT image of the cochlea of the inner ear using a bone algorithm

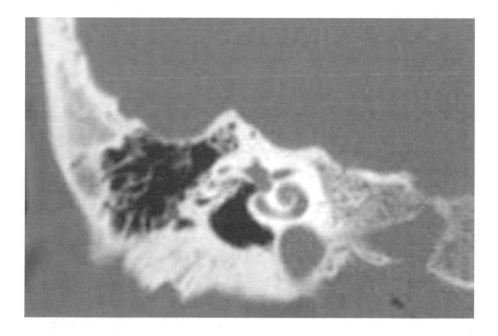

Figure 3.3b A computer generated (multiplanar reformatted) section showing the cochlea in a para-axial anatomical plane which illustrates the curls of the 'shell' which give it its name

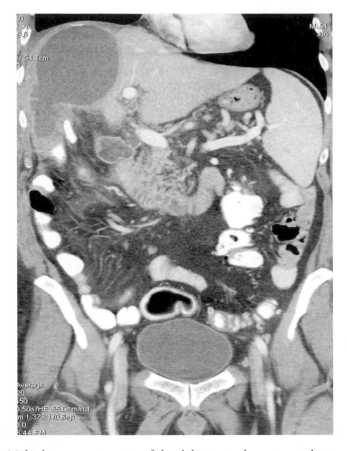

Figure 3.3c Multiplanar reconstruction of the abdomen to show a coronal view

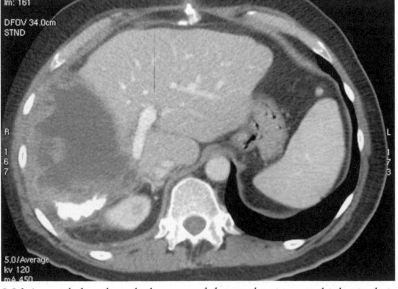

Figure 3.3d An axial slice through the upper abdomen showing a multi-density lesion in a patient's liver

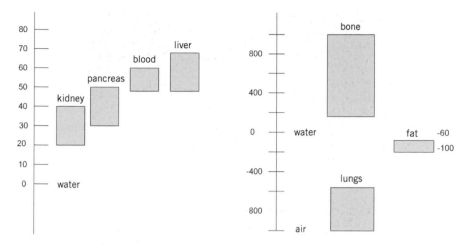

Figure 3.4 Diagram showing the typical Hounsfield unit values of body tissues and organs

Radiation dose and CT scanning

Radiation doses to the patient are relatively high for CT examinations (see Chapter 7) so it is essential that all health carers involved are aware of their responsibility to minimise the dose and to avoid irradiating pregnant patients wherever possible.

Case study

Rebecca (aged 33 years) had been referred for a CT of her abdomen as she had previously had a history of kidney stones. Before she was asked to get changed for the scan, Susan the radiographer asked her when her last period had begun. Rebecca told her that she was due to start menstruating the following day. Susan explained that because it was more than ten days after Rebecca's last period started, she could not have the test and it had to be deferred until a few days following the start of her next period. Rebecca was sent home and a new appointment was arranged within ten days of when her next period should start.

Technical note

CT is now considered the most appropriate imaging examination for the investigation of kidney stones as the scan can show a complete picture of the anatomy of the entire abdomen.

Unborn babies are particularly vulnerable to radiation-induced damage so, under normal circumstances, female patients between the ages of 11 and 55 years of age do not have CT scans of their abdomen or pelvis if there is a possibility of pregnancy or if they suspect that possibility.

Each department follows its own local guidelines about pregnancy checks and, if there is any doubt, the scan will not proceed unless the patient's life is at risk.

Patients may be alarmed and upset when the radiographer questions them about their periods and pregnancy status. Scans are sometimes deferred even if a patient's husband has had a vasectomy. Some departments will get a pregnancy test or request an ultrasound examination of the pelvis to ensure that there is no baby present if a patient has an uncertain menstrual history.

Procedures for requesting and accepting requests for CT scans and other medical imaging tests are discussed in more detail in Chapters 7 and 8, but with CT scans in particular, the examination should be limited to just the area of clinical concern and the scan **parameters** (see below) should be customised according to each individual patient's body shape and size. The area of the body to be scanned is decided by the radiologist – they choose the most appropriate **protocol** to follow and will determine whether or not contrast agents (see Chapter 2) and/or delayed imaging are required.

Health workers in the CT department only receive a radiation dose if they are participating in CT fluoroscopy as this involves them being in the scanning room while X-rays are generated. Normally hospital staff members will be in a CT **control room** where they will be separated from patients but can still see them through a lead-glass window (see Chapter 7). CT fluoroscopy is similar to general fluoroscopy (see Chapter 2) and is used when it is necessary to see the tip of a needle inserted into the body – perhaps to get a sample of tissue (biopsy), a sample of fluid (**aspiration**), or to drain a fluid build-up. Procedures done like this, under CT guidance, are safer and faster than if done in the operating theatre.

Originally, staff had to leave the CT scan room while a full exposure was made to locate needles. Now images can be obtained much faster, usually with a series of three short radiation pulses, and staff can remain in the room as the procedure time has been reduced significantly using this method. As in standard fluoroscopy staff dose can still be quite high, so personal radiation protection clothing, for example lead rubber aprons and thyroid shields (at least 0.35 mm lead equivalent), should be worn. Although patients can find it reassuring to have staff in the room the whole time during what can be an uncomfortable procedure, health care workers also need to remember to apply the **inverse square law** and take a step away from the gantry (the source of radiation) during the actual exposures.

It is the CT radiographer's responsibility to limit the radiation exposure dose by selecting optimal control settings. Most CT machines have an **automated exposure control** (AEC) which works out the optimum amount of radiation required depending upon the body size and shape. When the detectors have received enough radiation to generate an image of suitable quality the dose is reduced, then increased as a larger area passes through the scanner. AECs are designed to reduce patient dose and should be used for all abdominal and thoracic CT examinations where patient dose, for example to the thyroid and breast, is potentially the highest and may cause dose-related problems in later life (see Chapter 7). AECs are not used routinely for the brain as exposures to this area have to be consistent and comparable.

Many manufacturers are concentrating on technological improvements to reduce the radiation dose given that CT is the examination of choice for many common disorders.

The development of scanners

Early (first generation) scanners were slow and cumbersome – a ten slice brain scan could take up to an hour to obtain and display. This caused difficulty because it was almost impossible for patients to stay still for the five minutes it took to acquire the data for each section and any patient movement blurred the images. Image quality was also poor because the size of the **matrix** (the number of viewing elements in the image) was small, and therefore each **pixel** was a relatively large block of information and was easily visible within the image (see Figure 3.5a). In the early 1970s, matrix size was 80×80 pixels; today most scanners spread the image information over a matrix of 512×512 pixels, displaying a much clearer view of all areas (see Figure 3.5b).

Early CT scanning machines allowed little variation in the slice thickness as they acquired data in 10–13 mm sections, whereas now slices as thin as 0.5 mm are routinely acquired and the displayed images can be in single or multiples of this slice thickness.

As scanner design improved over time, the goal was to image in thin slices that would give the viewer more detailed anatomical information, i.e. better **spatial resolution**. However, even in the 1990s the dose to the patient had to be almost doubled if a reduction in the slice thickness by a half was required. Higher radiation doses had to be given for each slice to improve the **contrast resolution** and decrease electronic **noise** and streak

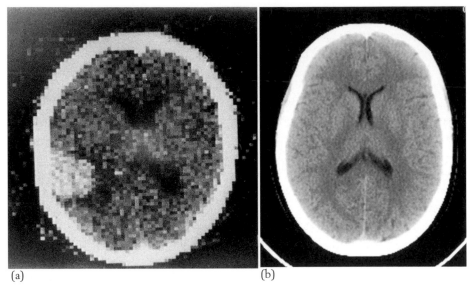

(a)   (b)

Figure 3.5 (a) Axial CT brain scan from 1974 (image reproduced with permission from the Medical Physics Dept at Ninewells Hospital, Dundee): (b) Modern day axial CT scan – normal appearance of the brain

artefact on the image. The most significant breakthrough was a change to continuous helical (spiral) scanning in 1989 (see Figure 3.6) – a development attributed to Willi Kalender who was working at Siemens (Kalender *et al.*, 1990). Kalender's new system had a single arc of detectors and an X-ray tube rotating in a helical fashion; at the same time the patient and the scanner table were moved at a pre-programmed speed through the gantry to allow a 'volume' rather than a 'slice' of data to be collected for each rotation of the X-ray tube. The resulting data could be reconstructed in any slice thickness with no additional radiation required. The reduced scanning time increased the number of patients who could be examined in a set period and also opened up the possibility of imaging disease processes using intravenous contrast agents more effectively. By using **contrast enhancement** and spiral CT in tandem, it became possible to distinguish arterial disease from venous since, in some diseases, abnorm-

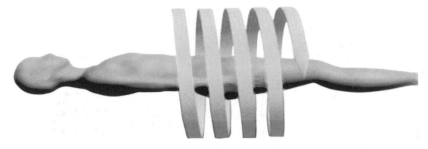

Figure 3.6 Schematic diagram showing helical X-ray tube movement with respect to the patient (image courtesy of GE Healthcare)

alities show up in the early arterial phase of contrast enhancement rather than the later venous phase. This enabled a more accurate evaluation and **staging** of major arterial diseases and vessel damage such as **aneurysm**.

At the turn of the twenty-first century, manufacturers introduced CT scanners with several banks of detectors side by side instead of in a single ring. This was possible by fixing the banks of detectors in the gantry and only moving the X-ray tube. This improved the speed of acquisition which, in turn, permitted even more manipulation of data. These 'multislice' CT (MSCT) scanners have the ability to create between four and 64 slices of information for a single rotation of the tube – and a single breath hold for the patient. Some manufacturers are still concentrating on making their scans even faster and it is anticipated that 256 slice units will be in clinical use from early 2008. MSCT has enabled scan acquisition times to be reduced from 5 s to 0.35 s, thus true functional almost 'real-time' CT is now possible using appropriate cardiac (heart) and angiographic (blood vessel) software packages (see Figures 3.7a, 3.7b and 3.7c).

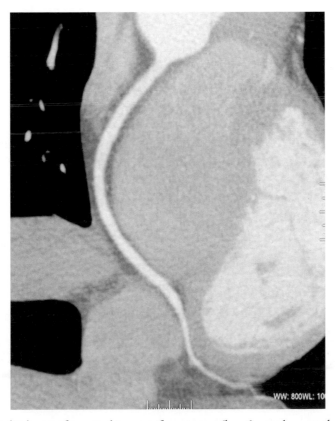

Figure 3.7a Multiplanar reformatted images of a coronary (heart) vessel – note that the entire heart was imaged in 5.2 seconds

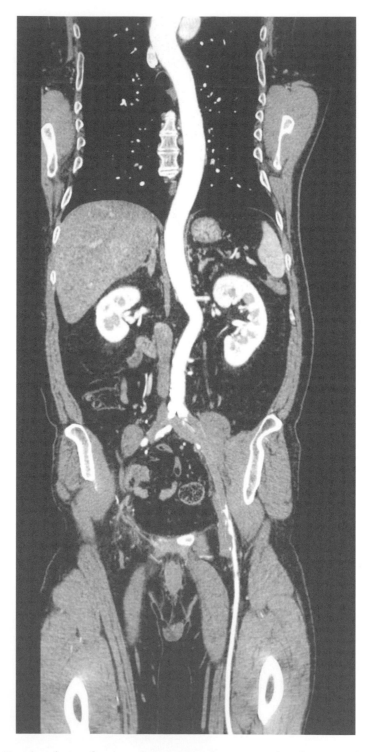

Figure 3.7b Vessel analysis software package used to demonstrate that this patient has severe vascular disease where the main blood vessel of the abdomen – the aorta – splits into two to supply the legs

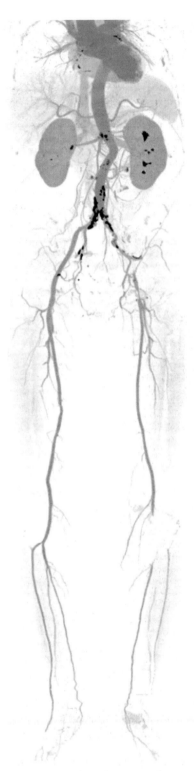

Figure 3.7c Computer reconstruction using an alternate software package which separates out just the blood supply information (image courtesy of GE Healthcare)

Factors affecting image quality

Controlling the quality of the CT image is highly complex but the principle is that thinner slices generally have better spatial resolution. Technology has improved so much that high quality images can now be obtained with very little increase in radiation dose or examination time and thin slices (0.5 mm) can be used routinely. The radiographer can alter several scan parameters to improve how the images appear.

Case study

Susan, an experienced CT radiographer, was explaining to Sam, a newly qualified member of staff, what factors should be altered throughout the scan to get the best images.

- **Slice thickness** – thin slices give better spatial resolution.

- **X-ray tube current** (mAs) – controls the amount of radiation generated by the X-ray tube during scanning: generally larger patients require higher mAs values. Some body areas require more mAs so that the image will have less noise and soft tissues structures in the body will be better displayed.

- **FoV** – the 'field of view' controls the amount of the body that is shown on the viewing screen: the larger the body area appears on the screen, the more information the reader will have.

- **Filter/algorithm** – Susan explained that computer software programs control how the images are reconstructed and that, for instance, a filter or **algorithm** can be used to 'sharpen' the image, particularly when imaging bony structures such as the inner ear or **fractures**.

- **Pitch of acquisition** – this is the speed of the table movement (mms^{-1}) proportional to the slice thickness (mm) during helical CT scanning. Higher pitch values (faster movement) generally result in poorer image quality but expose the patient to less radiation. Susan explained how the choice of pitch level is specific to each individual examination and patient and involves her assessing the patient's size, the degree of detail required in the images and the need for multiplanar reconstructions. She then explained that she had to balance all these factors against the radiation dose involved, in order to select the appropriate pitch. Sam said that she knew that 3rd generation scanners usually used a pitch of one, but that nowadays most MSCT scanners used a pitch between 1.2 and 1.7 to give the best quality image for the lowest radiation dose.

A radiographer uses algorithms to choose how to view the image. By **windowing** the image (manipulating the viewing data by changing the **grey-scale** allocation across the range of HU values in the image), it is possible to display small density differences that might otherwise be missed. Windowing allows the different appearances of soft tissue and bony structures to be shown for the same data slice without examining, and thus irradiating, the patient twice (see Figure 3.8a, 3.8b and 3.8c).

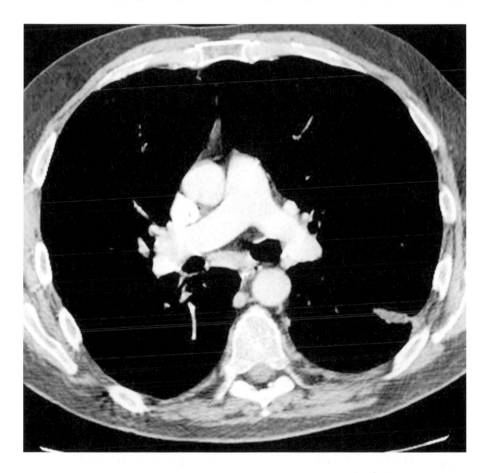

Figure 3.8a Axial section through the chest using a soft tissue filter/algorithm to show intravenous contrast in the vessels taking blood from the heart to the lungs – note that the black areas represent lung tissue

HAVING A CT SCAN

As an illustration, let us consider a patient having one of the most common CT examinations – a scan of the abdomen.

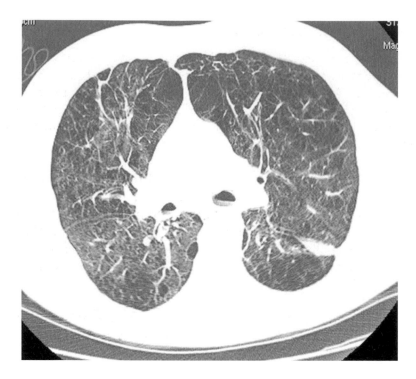

Figure 3.8b Same axial section as in 3.8a, but reconstructed using a 'lung' algorithm and displayed at different viewing window levels to show the anatomical detail in the lung tissue

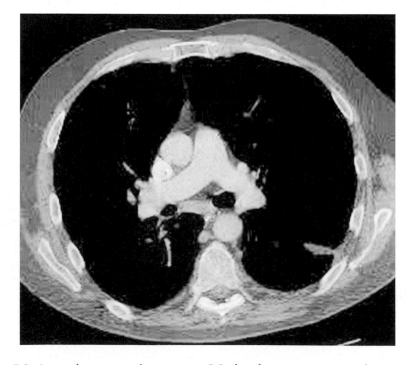

Figure 3.8c Again, the same axial section as in 3.8a, but this time reconstructed using a 'bone' algorithm and viewed on a wide window setting to make the bone detail sharper

Preparing for a ct examination

For many CT examinations, no special preparation is required. However, most patients are asked not to eat anything for at least four hours before attending for a CT of the abdomen and chest. This is because any food in the stomach may be mistaken for disease and also because patients who have starved are less likely to feel nauseous if a contrast agent has to be injected.

As in conventional radiography, some soft tissue structures can be seen and differentiated on CT images because of their different radiation attenuation properties, while others have very similar attenuation properties and any resultant differences in greyscale values allocated to the digital image are too small to be noticeable. In such cases, the density of structures can be artificially altered by giving the patient a contrast agent (see Table 3.1).

As described in Chapter 2, sometimes the **lumen** (channel) or cavity of a hollow body structure is filled with a contrast agent so that its walls show up well.

Positive contrast agents can be given by mouth, by intravenous injection, or by direct introduction into a body cavity, e.g. the back passage (per rectum) or a fistula (abnormal opening into the body from the outside), but patients are often also asked not to pass water before a CT scan because urine in the bladder is a good natural negative contrast agent.

Case study

When Bryony arrived in the CT department an hour before her scan as her appointment letter had requested, she was a bit startled to be given a jug of liquid that tasted of orange and aniseed by Angela the health care assistant, who asked her to drink a glass every ten minutes. Angela explained that about half a litre was needed to fill Bryony's stomach, so that the walls would be stretched thin and that up to one litre was needed to fill the small bowel. She explained that an even distribution of contrast agent in the small bowel would help the radiologist pick up any abnormalities and tell the difference between the bowel and lymph nodes and blood vessels close by. Although it didn't taste too bad, drinking so much felt rather daunting. Angela explained that if they had been looking lower in her large bowel (colon) or rectum, a longer period of preparation would have been required and Bryony would have needed some of the contrast agent 12 hours in advance.

Contrast type	Contrast agent	Method of administration	CT Applications	CT Protocols	Notes	Alerts
Positive looks white on images	Barium sulphate suspension 96%	Orally	Re-staging examinations, where a patient has a diagnosis and has had surgery; First scans	Up to one litre taken gradually over an hour	Less dense than that used for barium meals and enemas (see Chapter 2)	Never injected; Not given if a bowel leak (perforation) is suspected
	Water-soluble iodine preparation	Orally	As above; Depending upon local protocols	3% concentration in water; Up to 1 litre taken gradually over an hour	It is assumed that substances that are safe to inject are also safe to eat	Check for allergies required – see Chapter 2
		Rectally	Used in patients where pelvic disease is suspected.	Sent to the patient's home in small ampoules 10 mls to be taken 12 hours before the scan		Clear instructions must be sent with the substance to ensure that the patient has no allergy
			To fill the lower large bowel and rectum	3% concentration in warm water; 100 mls introduced per rectum via a thick rubber catheter		
			Used when we need to define rectum following an initial scan	Hand injection, 50 mls		
		Intravenous injection	Used in almost all cases of thorax and abdomen and when vessels and organ function is required	By pump, 100 mls at three mls per second	Requires a check that the patient's kidneys are functioning well	Must ensure that the patient has no iodine allergy
Negative Looks dark grey on images	Water	Orally	New staging of stomach and oesophagus tumours; Large and small bowel diseases	Up to one litre taken gradually over an hour		Never injected
	Air or carbon dioxide	Rectally	Used for CT colonography to inflate the large bowel	Difficult to measure, but four litres of carbon dioxide is usual		Care should be taken not to over-inflate the bowel in case of perforation
No Prep			Some departments use no preparation for abdomens for trauma as they believe it may cause difficulty when/if the patient is taken to the operating theatre and given an anaesthetic			

Table 3.1 Contrast agent use in CT

Technical note

Contrast agents can be either negative with a low HU value, such as water, which gives a dark-grey appearance in the image, or positive, such as water-soluble iodine preparations which have higher HU values and appear white in the image (see Figure 3.9a and b).

Usually negative agents are used for the food pipe (oesophagus) and stomach where small abnormalities need to be clearly seen to stage a cancer. However, many CT centres are now using water as a contrast agent for many different scans so you can't assume that its use means the scan is for cancer.

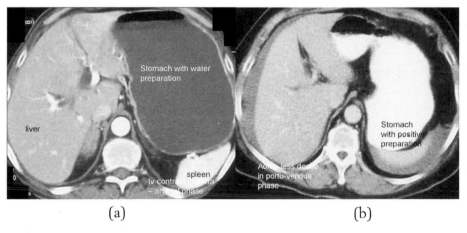

(a)   (b)

Figure 3.9 (a) Axial section through the upper abdomen showing water in the stomach (dark grey) and intravenous contrast in the aorta (bright white). The liver is not as bright as the spleen because the contrast has not yet filled all of the vascular spaces in the liver. (b) In this axial section of the upper abdomen, the stomach is very bright because the patient was given a positive contrast agent preparation to drink beforehand. The liver is also brighter because this scan slice was obtained 30 seconds later than the image on the left

At the start of the CT examination, the patient is asked to lie on their back on the CT table so that a **scanogram** image can be taken (see Figure 3.10). For this, the X-ray tube remains underneath the patient, to keep the radiation dose to sensitive organs such as the thyroid and breast low as the table moves through the gantry. The scanogram image is similar to a conventional radiograph and should include all the areas of the body to be examined during the scan; it is used to check that the patient is correctly positioned. The radiographer then uses the computer to mark lines on the image to show the levels at which the computer will start and stop collecting data during the scan. Once the radiographer has programmed the pitch of acquisition and selected the speed of intra-venous contrast agent injection, if it is to be used, the scanner is activated and the co-ordinated X-ray detector rotation, table movement and contrast injection begin.

Once all the scan data have been collected, the radiographer looks at the images on the viewing monitor to decide if enough information is available for a diagnosis or whether additional scans are needed.

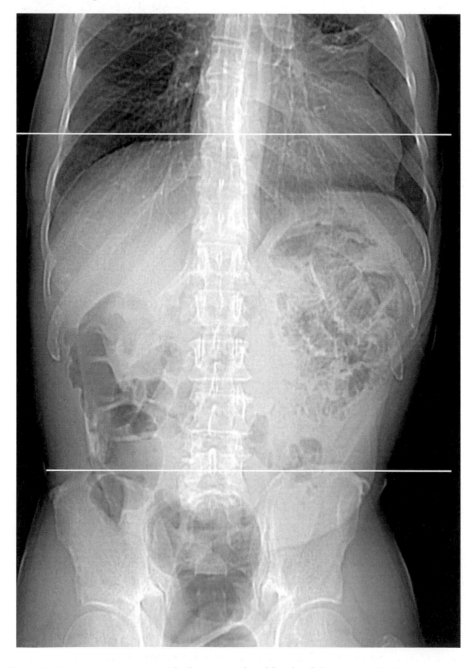

Figure 3.10 Scanogram image with the start and end levels of the scan marked up

Case study

Once the data had been collected for Bryony's abdominal CT images, Sam, the radiographer, looked at them to check that the contrast agents had shown up all the necessary anatomy. Sam noticed that the oral contrast agent had not completely filled one or two of the small bowel loops in the pelvis and that there was one area not showing up well (see Figure 3.11). Susan, the senior CT radiographer, explained that Sam could either ask Bryony to drink some more fluid to 'push' the contrast agent through or could ask Bryony to wait a while and then take some more slices.

Technical note

Additional slice acquisition and delayed scanning are sometimes needed if blood vessels, or an organ lumen or cavity, do not appear to have filled properly. It does not necessarily mean that an abnormality has been seen, thus patients need not be concerned if further slices are performed.

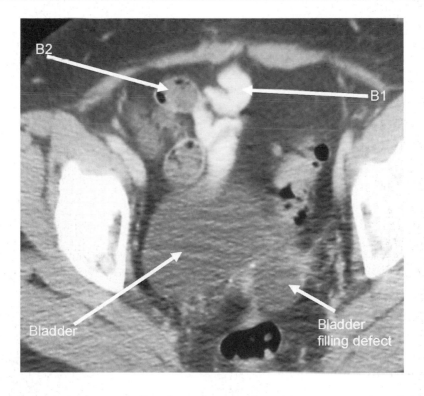

Figure 3.11 Axial CT section through a pelvis: some bowel loops (B1) are distended with positive contrast agent (lighter shades of grey) while others (B2) remain unfilled and appear darker. More contrast agent or delayed scanning is required so that these can be observed when full to ensure that there is no underlying disease

Intravenous contrast agents are given to patients having CT scans when the tissues that need to be demonstrated do not communicate with the bowel, e.g. an artery passing through a muscle, or when small tumours may have HU values very close to those of the surrounding organ.

Case study

Paul arrived for a scan of his pancreas (the insulin producing gland in the upper abdomen) just as Susan, the CT radiographer, had finished looking at the request card that his consultant had sent to the imaging department. Unfortunately, Paul's consultant suspected that he might have a tumour. Susan had chosen a **dual-phase** scan protocol to show this best and explained to Paul that he had to keep very still when the table was moving during the scan. Susan also asked Paul to hold his breath during the scan to help keep his internal organs still as well. Once Paul understood what he had to do, Susan connected the contrast agent injection pump to a vein at the front of Paul's elbow and then went into the CT control room to start the image acquisition process. Susan had been careful to reassure Paul that, although in the past patients often felt sick when large quantities of contrast agents were injected, this was unusual with modern contrast agents and that all he was likely to feel was a warm 'glow' – particularly in his pelvic area.

Clinical insight

Dual-phase scans can be used for many reasons besides looking for cancers, but in this case it was used first to image just the pancreas during the arterial phase of contrast enhancement so that any subtle and early changes in blood supply could be seen – tumours usually have an increased blood supply compared with normal tissue. The second phase of the scan covered all the upper abdomen, from the top of the diaphragm to the lowermost tip of the liver (and included the tail of the pancreas in the upper left corner of the abdomen), and collected data while the contrast agent was in the portal veins. This second phase is useful for showing any secondary (**metastatic**) tumours in the liver.

Each radiology department has a different CT workload, depending on whether it is in a district general hospital, a teaching hospital or a tertiary (specialist) referral centre. Although the exact patient mix varies greatly from one department to another, overall approximately 40 per cent of CT patients seen are for brain scanning, of which only approximately 15 per cent require an intravenous contrast agent injection compared to approximately 80 per cent of patients seen who are having CT scans for neck, chest and abdominal problems.

For brain disorders the contrast agent can be injected by hand, but for most CT scans almost all hospitals now use automatic injectors programmed to deliver a set volume of contrast agent at a specific flow rate. The exact volume and flow rate will depend on the pathology being investigated, but for a typical CT abdominal scan 100 ml are delivered at 3 ml per second. The contrast agent injection is co-ordinated with the CT scan data acquisition and often includes a time delay after the injection begins and before scanning starts to allow the contrast agent to get from the injection site to the organs of interest. Delays of 25 s – 75 s are often used, depending on the abnormality suspected, the speed of the scanner, and the diameters of the vein and needle being used for the injection.

Case study

Once Susan had completed the dual-phase scan, Sam noticed a **lesion** in Paul's liver. Dr Jones, the radiologist, explained that because it had a low density centre, measuring more than 10 HU, it was unlikely to be just a simple cyst and could be a metastasis. Dr Jones asked Sam to wait a few moments and then feed the scan table back into the scanner and take a few more slices just at the level of the lesion. After this time delay, the lesion had filled completely with the contrast agent and Dr Jones was now more sure that it was a secondary tumour deposit. If the lesion had maintained a low HU measurement they would have concluded that it was more likely to be a benign cyst. Without the delayed CT imaging, Paul might have had to come back to the imaging department at a later date for an ultrasound (see Chapter 5) or an MRI (see Chapter 6) scan to further **stage** his disease.

Technical note

Re-scanning at a different time after contrast agent injection will show the organs and lesions at different stages of contrast enhancement – since organs and tumours fill with contrast agents at different rates this can help the doctors decide exactly what type of tumour the lesion is likely to be – a haemangioma (benign blood vessel tumour) in the liver can take up to five minutes to fill (Caseiro-Alves et al., 2007) whereas a secondary cancer (metastasis) enhances much more quickly.

Once all the required data have been collected, patients can go home or back to the ward; the radiographer will generate any necessary multi-planar reformatted images before the examination is formally reported, usually by the radiologist.

WHEN IS CT A USEFUL TEST?

For many years, patients attending different hospitals did not get the same diagnostic investigations and this led to different standards of patient care across the country – the so-called 'postcode lottery'. In several areas of medical practice this has now been addressed by bodies such as the National Institute for Health and Clinical Excellence (NICE) and there are some national referral standards such as, for example, for head injury and stroke patients (NICE 2001, 2003a, 2007). For other clinical conditions, although there are no fixed national guidelines, CT practice is nevertheless reasonably standardised across the country, with professional bodies such as the Royal College of Radiologists providing guidelines for initial staging scans for patients with cancer, for example (RCR, 2006).

Case study

Dr Jones, the radiologist, had noticed a small dense lesion in the right middle lobe of Edward's lung during a routine chest X-ray. Dr Jones knew that there were some 'cancer guidelines' that recommended that Edward should be sent straight back to his GP with his chest X-ray report containing instructions to refer him to hospital urgently (NICE 2005). Dr Jones could then arrange an urgent CT scan to confirm a cancer diagnosis and to stage Edward's disease accurately.

Technical note

Most imaging of cancer patients is now driven by government guidelines and targets that ensure timely examination and reporting as part of nationally determined standard treatment plans – this helps to ensure patients have the same standard of diagnosis and treatment wherever they live throughout the UK.

Head injury

Following a head injury, a person is at risk of having a blood clot in or around their brain (intracranial haematoma). Although some of these patients will need surgery to prevent irreversible brain damage, most people who attend hospital with a history of head injury are at low risk of this. The NICE recommends that people who attend Accident and Emergency departments with acute head injury should be assessed by a doctor within 15 minutes of their arrival in hospital (NICE, 2007). The recommendations also explain which patients should be referred for head CT and the timescales within which this should be performed – some scans need to be done within an hour of a request being received in the radiology department (NICE, 2003a; NICE, 2007). In order to comply with this requirement, most centres have radiologists available 24 hours a day, seven days a week, to interpret head scans: sometimes this is via a home-hospital computer network link – an example of **telemedicine**.

Stroke

Hospitals that treat patients who have just had a **stroke** should be able to perform head CT within three hours of it occurring in order that treatment with **thrombolytic** (clot dissolving) agents can be started within this time window if appropriate. This requirement puts an additional strain on radiology services since a CT radiographer has to stay in the hospital overnight and at weekends to provide this service (RCP, 2004).

Cancer

CT is widely used to diagnose and stage cancer. Cancer staging involves determining the extent and severity of the disease – whether it is confined to one location in the body (the **primary** site), whether it has spread to other structures close by (local spread), or has spread to distant parts of the body (secondary sites or metastases). Accurate staging is critical for both the patient and their health carers so they can choose which treatment is likely to have the best chance of controlling or curing the disease. CT is also a good investigation for checking if a tumour has been removed completely or to see how well it is responding to treatment.

Acute medical and surgical cases

Specially designated hospital wards that receive patients directly from home or from their GPs, known as medical and surgical admissions units, rely on a fast service from radiology departments, especially for CT scans, so that they can establish a diagnosis, treat and/or discharge patients as quickly as possible. CT is an ideal test for patients with sudden onset abdominal pain – often conventional radiography is not performed when doctors suspect that a patient's problem is due to a blockage in the bowel (obstruction) or appendicitis. These patients are likely to be sent for a confirmatory CT scan and then straight to the operating theatre.

It is not unusual for patients admitted to hospital with severe headaches to have an immediate CT scan – if a doctor considers a patient to be **stable** and the CT scan is 'negative' many such patients can be sent home after a short period of observation, in the confidence that there is no serious brain abnormality.

Trauma

CT is an important diagnostic test for assessing the damage caused when people have major accidents. Depending on access and local expertise, patients with severe abdomen and chest injuries may be referred for CT or may have an initial ultrasound in the trauma room. Although CT involves moving the patient away from the Accident and Emergency department and getting them onto the CT table, it is a more sensitive test for locating small amounts of free fluid in the abdomen or pelvis (Benya *et al.*, 2000). Free fluid may indicate that a blood vessel has burst or is leaking, or that an organ has ruptured or been pierced – when free fluid is detected in a critically ill patient they usually need to have an operation as soon as possible.

CT will detect more fractures than can be seen on conventional radiographs and also allows the damage to the soft tissue structures close by to be assessed at the same time. MSCT and MPR can be used to obtain detailed images of severe fractures prior to surgery.

Less serious soft tissue and bone injuries are often first examined with ultrasound or conventional radiography respectively (RCR, 2007). Ultrasound does not have any radiation dose and plain radiography should be used where a diagnosis is likely to be obtained at a lower dose than is involved in a CT examination. While local protocols for referral should exist in most hospitals, if in doubt nurses and doctors in the trauma department should seek guidance from radiologists and radiographers in order that they can request the most appropriate examinations and techniques.

Advanced CT applications

Although it has not altered the basic principles of disease management, advanced software has opened up new areas of application for CT. Most notably, vascular and vessel analysis (cardiac and angiographic) packages allow review of the initial data collected about aneurysms or tortuous vessels in any anatomical plane and these are now commonly used to plan vascular surgery (Kessel and Robertson, 2005) and for routine post-surgical imaging of **stents** and other therapeutic devices (see Chapter 2).

Display of images in 3D format can be used, in particular, to demonstrate bone fragments – few complex fractures are now operated on without the prior use of 3D MPR CT scans. These techniques are also invaluable in other clinical specialities where a knowledge of three-dimensional anatomy is required, e.g. assessing complex spinal deformities. **Virtual surgery** can be performed on 3D data sets to simulate the removal of parts of the body and to model the predicted results of a reconstructive operation. The CT software can even be used to create real 3D models, for example for patients with facial deformities or those requiring complex joint replacements, so that 'experimental' surgery can be performed on the model prior to attempting the real thing on the patient.

One of the most widely used recent advances in CT software is virtual colonoscopy – known as CT colonography (CTC). During this technique, the large bowel (colon) is filled with either air or carbon dioxide to such a degree that the computer can reconstruct images along the lumen as if it were being visualised from within (see Figure 3.12). Research studies are currently underway to compare CT colonography with conventional **colonoscopy** (where a small camera on a tube is placed into the colon via the rectum) and barium enema (see Chapter 2) to see which test is best for locating and monitoring pre-cancerous tumours known as **polyps**.

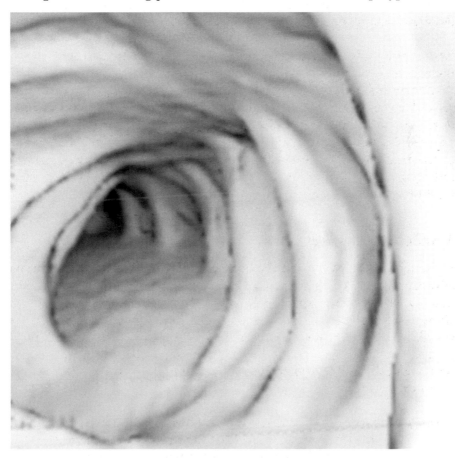

Figure 3.12 An image of the large bowel reconstructed from a CT colonography examination. The inside of the colon looks like an underground cavern – the dependent fluid seen in the 'floor of the cave' is bowel content that did not get cleaned out with the pre-examination laxatives

SUMMARY

To a large extent, government targets now shape hospital CT services and national guidelines exist to indicate when it is the most appropriate test. It is the test of choice for several medical conditions because it can minimise the time from patient presentation to getting an accurate and complete diagnosis. Although CT is the optimal investigation for many chest, abdomen and brain problems and is a useful examination for people with cancer, its relatively high radiation dose should not be forgotten whenever a referral is made – sometimes techniques with no or lower radiation dose should be performed in the first instance.

Heavy reliance on computer software in CT scanning means that it is becoming increasingly complex; this requires more and more sophisticated operator and interpreter skill. The extended use of tele-communication networking is also allowing out-of-hours services to grow, with radiologists now able to access and report emergency cases at home without having to attend the hospital – this should help make rapid access to 24-hour CT services a clinical reality.

FURTHER READING

Chapman, S. and Nakielney, R. (2001) *A Guide to Radiological Procedures* (4th Ed). Edinburgh: Saunders
An informative guide to examinations carried out in a radiology department. Useful for those wanting to know a little more about radiology.

Hofer, M. (2000) *CT Teaching Manual.* New York: Thieme
A very readable manual for students working in CT in a radiology department. Gives a good in-depth understanding of CT and teaches cross-sectional anatomy. The quiz questions are also useful.

Martin, J. and Sutton, D.G. (2006) *Practical Radiation Protection in Health Care.* Oxford: Oxford University Press
A useful book explaining all aspects of radiation protection in detail. For those students who want to know more about dose measurement and safety factors.

Seeram, E. (2001) *Computed Tomography: Physical Principles, Clinical Applications and Quality Control* (2nd Ed). Philadelphia: Saunders
Much more physics based, but well worth reading for the more seriously interested.

Chapter 4

Radionuclide Imaging (Scintigraphy)
Fiona Ware

INTRODUCTION

The aim of this chapter is to increase your awareness and understanding of how radionuclide imaging (or scintigraphy as it is also known) works and how it is commonly used in medical imaging. After an explanation of how scintigraphic images are generated, routine clinical applications of the technique will be described to give an overview of what it involves for the person being investigated, how the images are used to look at how the body works and any changes that might be **pathological**, and how scintigraphic data can be quantified to measure changes in organ **physiology** (function). Finally, the latest developments in scintigraphic imaging are discussed.

PRINCIPLES OF RADIONUCLIDE IMAGING/SCINTIGRAPHY

Radionuclide imaging (RNI)/scintigraphy (usually undertaken in a Nuclear Medicine department) is a medical imaging technique that involves the introduction of a **radioactive** substance into the body. As the substance undergoes **radioactive decay** radiation is emitted and can be picked up by a radiation detection device placed outside the body close to the skin surface. As most of the emitted radiation is in the form of **gamma rays** (see Chapter 1) the detection device is known as a **gamma camera** (see Figure 4.1). The gamma camera is linked to a computer system that allows images to be stored, manipulated and displayed in digital format. As with other digital imaging techniques, images can be archived onto a *PACS* or other electronic medium, can be viewed as **soft copy** on a TV monitor, or can be printed out as **hard copy** on photographic paper or conventional radiographic film (see Chapter 1).

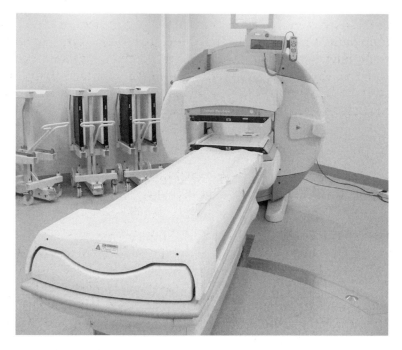

Figure 4.1 A modern dual-headed gamma camera and patient examination couch

Radiopharmaceuticals

The radioactive substances used in scintigraphy are composed of a radio-active element (the **radionuclide**) that is 'labelled' (chemically attached) to a pharmaceutical product. The pharmaceutical products are drugs that have been designed to 'target' specific functional processes in the body so that they pass through, and sometimes accumulate in, a particular organ or bodily system. Together the radionuclide and pharmaceutical preparation is known as a **radiopharmaceutical** or **radiotracer**. A list of commonly used radiopharmaceuticals is given in Table 4.1.

Clinical application	Radionuclide	Pharmaceutical label
Bone scintigraphy	Tc99m	HDP (hydroxymethylene diphosphonate)
Lung (V) ventilation	Tc99m	DTPA (Diethylene triamine pentaacetic acid)
Lung (V) ventilation	Kr81m gas	not applicable
Lung (Q) perfusion	Tc99m	MAA (macroaggregated albumin)
Renal scintigraphy	Tc99m	MAG3 (mercaptoacetyltriglycine)
Myocardial SPECT	Tc99m	MIBI (sestamibi)
PET-CT	F18	FDG (fluorodeoxyglucose)

Table 4.1 Commonly used radiopharmaceuticals

Most radiopharmaceuticals are administered by injecting them into a vein in the patient's arm (intravenous injection), but some are administered orally (swallowed/ingested) into the digestive system and some are inhaled as vapour using an aerosol device or a face mask. Radiopharmaceuticals are well tolerated by adults and children alike and are most unlikely to cause any unpleasant side effects.

Case study

Sally, the radiographer, was scheduled to work in the hospital radiopharmacy for the week. She knew that this would involve preparing fresh radiopharmaceuticals each day and that she would have to do this under **aseptic conditions** (using sterile equipment and wearing special clothing and surgical gloves). By mid-morning on Monday, she had drawn up all the individual injections, making sure they were carefully labelled for each patient who had an appointment that day. She took them to the Nuclear Medicine department in a lead shielded box where they were stored ready for use.

Technical note

Radiopharmaceuticals generally have a very short 'shelf' life, which is why patients must keep quite strictly to their appointment times so that their own individual radiopharmaceutical injection can be used at the right time to give the best quality images.

The time between introducing the radiopharmaceutical into the body and its arrival in the anatomical area of interest depends on its route of administration and the physiological process of its **uptake** and excretion (removal from the body). If injected intravenously the preparation is transported around the body in the **systemic circulation** ensuring rapid delivery. Once it arrives at the organ, or in the system to be examined, the pharmaceutical 'label' is recognised and the radiotracer is actively removed from the blood as part of a natural physiological process. Radiopharmaceutical uptake may be relatively slow, for instance in bone, or very rapid, for example in the kidneys or heart; patient positioning near the gamma camera has to be timed accordingly.

Radionuclides

The mostly commonly used radionuclide in diagnostic scintigraphy is Technetium 99m (Tc99m). Tc99m can be obtained at a relatively low cost on a daily basis within a hospital using a generator system (see Figure 4.2a and b). The generator contains the 'parent' radionuclide Molybdenum 99 (Mo99), which decays continuously to produce the 'daughter'

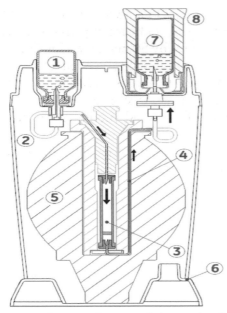

1 Eluent – 0.9% saline solution

2 Tubing linking eluent to chromatographic column

3 Chromatographic column – contains parent nuclide Mo-99 on an inert carrier, (alumina)

4 Needle linking column to evacuated glass vial

5 Thick lead shielding

6 Tough plastic casing

7 Evacuated glass vial – receives eluate containing Tc99m from column

8 Collection vial shield.

Figure 4.2a Schematic diagram of the inside of a Mo99-Tc99m radionuclide generator (illustration courtesy of GE Healthcare)

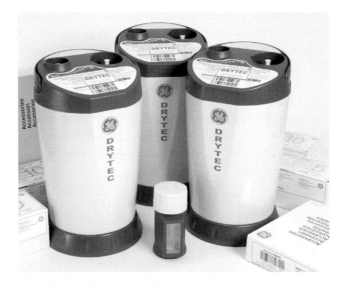

Figure 4.2b Commercially available Mo99-Tc99m generator and accessories (image courtesy of GE Healthcare)

product Tc99m. Tc99m has many characteristics that make it suitable for medical imaging:

- it combines readily with a variety of pharmaceuticals;
- it emits only gamma rays;
- it has a short physical **half-life**.

All radioactive substances decay naturally to a non-radioactive state; the half-life is the time taken for the amount of radioactivity present in a given volume of radiopharmaceutical to reduce by 50 per cent – for Tc99m this is six hours. Radionuclides with a long half-life remain active for an extended period in the body and result in higher radiation doses to the patient; with too short a half-life the radionuclide might not remain active in the body for long enough to emit sufficient radiation to create adequate images. With a half-life of six hours, Tc99m allows the radiation dose to the patient to be kept as low as reasonably possible while still obtaining images of good diagnostic quality.

Image acquisition

Once the radiopharmaceutical has been administered to the patient, image acquisition may start immediately (dynamic study) or may occur after a specific time interval (static study) depending on the type of examination being performed.

In dynamic studies, image acquisition starts as soon as an intravenous injection has been given to ensure that accurate data are collected about organ function. In renal scintigraphy (radionuclide imaging of the kidneys – see below) for example, the radiotracer is extracted from the blood and may be excreted by the kidneys within 15 minutes.

In a static study such as bone scintigraphy, image acquisition begins after a delay of two to three hours following injection of the radiopharmaceutical. This allows time for a sufficient amount of the radiotracer to be taken up in the bony **skeleton** – bone **metabolism** being a much slower process than renal **perfusion**.

The gamma camera

The gamma camera is a specially designed radiation detector with a large **field of view**. It contains a sodium iodide crystal that absorbs gamma radiation photons emitted by the radionuclide inside a patient. The gamma photon energy is then converted into light energy within the sodium iodide crystal by a process known as scintillation. Scintillations (tiny light flashes) are converted into electronic signals and amplified within the gamma camera. The gamma camera co-ordinates scintillation events with their relative spatial location and the electronic signals are stored on a **digital image matrix** in a way that represents the position of the radionuclide within the body.

The radionuclide image is built up over time as hundreds of thousands of scintillation events, known as 'counts', are detected and captured. Each 'count' represents a single gamma **photon** that has reached the sodium iodide crystal and caused it to scintillate. The scintigraphic image is displayed as a 'matrix of dots', with each dot representing a pulse of scintillations from each gamma photon (see Figure 4.3). For static imaging, 'counts' are acquired continually until enough have been collected to produce a recognisable image – in adults counts between 500 and 800,000 are required depending on the particular examination being performed. The static image is essentially an 'anatomical representation' of the physiology of an organ that is viewed and assessed for **pathological** change.

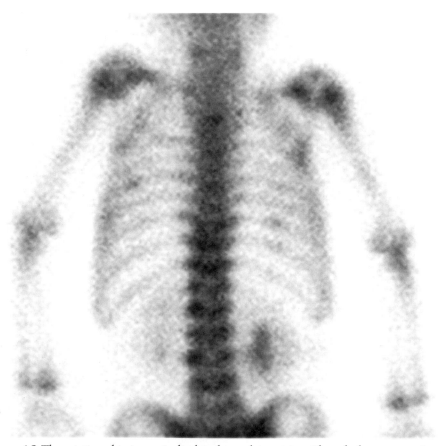

Figure 4.3 The scintigraphic image is displayed as a dot matrix with each dot representing a single scintillation

Since radionuclide images are built up over time, the data can also be analysed to show how the radioactivity level within an organ changes with time; this is known as dynamic imaging and gives additional useful information about changes in organ physiology/function. Essentially, sequential 'frames' of static image data are acquired and then viewed in rapid succession; individual frame times can vary from one to 60 seconds. The analysis and display of dynamic imaging data may be either qualitative (visual) or in quantitative (numerical) format. Sequential image frames may be viewed in rapid succession as a cine/video loop, or the data may be converted into a graph called a **time-activity curve** (see Figure 4.4). Quantitative analysis involves taking measurements and making calculations from the time-activity curve data (see 'renal scintigraphy' later in this chapter).

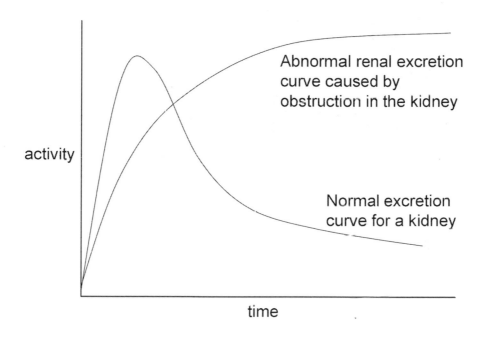

Figure 4.4 Radionuclide time-activity curves

The ability to quantify function helps to gauge the severity of a disease process. This can help doctors choose the most appropriate course of treatment for each particular patient and it also helps them monitor if patients are deteriorating (getting worse) or improving (getting better) by comparing measurements from similar examinations performed on different dates.

Radiation protection

The medical use of radiopharmaceuticals is governed by MARS 1978 and ARSAC (Administration of Radioactive Substances Advisory Committe) Legislation also obliges health care workers to protect themselves (IRR 1999) and their patients (IR(ME) R2000) from unnecessary radiation hazards. As with all medical investigations involving **ionising radiation**, the potential benefits of performing scintigraphy must outweigh its risks (see Chapter 7). Patients will typically get a higher radiation dose from an RNI investigation compared with a general radiograph, but doses associated with scintigraphy are significantly less than those associated with computed tomography (CT) scans (see Table 4.2 and Table 4.3).

Diagnostic imaging investigation	Typical effective dose (mSv)	Approximate equivalent duration of natural background radiation (UK average)
Chest radiograph	0.02	3 days
Lung perfusion scintigraphy (Tc99m)	1	6 months
Computed tomography – chest	8	3.6 years

Table 4.2 Comparative radiation doses for investigations of the chest (RCR, 2007)

Area of the body (all Tc99m)	Typical effective dose (mSv)	Approximate equivalent duration of natural background radiation (UK average)
Lung (perfusion) Kidneys Thyroid	1	6 months
Bone	4	1.8 years
Cardiac SPECT	8	3.6 years
PET-CT (tumour imaging)	8	3.6 years

Table 4.3 Comparative radiation doses for RNI investigations (RCR, 2007; ARSAC, 2006)

The most important radiation protection measure is a properly completed and signed **referral** for each patient. In the context of RNI examinations, the referral acts as the legal prescription for the radiopharmaceutical and ensures that each patient receives the correct radiotracer preparation and correct dose. Accurate information about the patient's age, weight and clinical condition is needed to ensure that an appropriate investigation has been requested and so the examination can be **justified**. Inappropriate RNI investigations expose both patients and staff to radiation unnecessarily.

Radiation protection for patients

Once a radiopharmaceutical has been administered to a patient, they become radioactive for a short time; the duration of this depends on the type and amount of radiopharmaceutical used. Most radiopharmaceuticals are eliminated from the body via the kidneys and bladder, so it is important that patients are able to pass urine properly or that they have a bladder catheter inserted. Patients are encouraged to drink plenty of fluid and to empty their bladder frequently after an RNI examination; increasing the amount and frequency of urine being passed helps flush residual active radiopharmaceutical from the body more quickly and thus minimises the radiation dose to the patient.

Generally, for most routine scintigraphic procedures, there will be no need to place any restriction on patient movement or proximity to others once they have left the department. Following some RNI investigations however, Nuclear Medicine department staff will occasionally advise patients to avoid prolonged physical contact with pregnant women and children for varied periods of time depending on the scan.

Case study

Amanda arrived in the Nuclear Medicine Department for her lung scan. She was a bit anxious as she had just established a breast feeding routine with her son Mikey, who had been born just a few days ago. Sally checked Amanda's name, date of birth and address details and then asked Amanda to confirm that she had recently given birth and asked whether she was breast or bottle feeding her baby.

When Amanda said she was breast feeding, Sally explained that she would have to stop breast feeding for 14 hours after having the lung scan radionuclide injection. Sally also advised Amanda to express and discard her breast milk and avoid 'cuddling' Mikey for long periods during this 14-hour restriction period. Amanda was told she could re-start her usual breast feeding routine at the end of this time.

Technical note

Tc99mMAA, the radionuclide used for lung scintigraphy, can be secreted in breast milk. New mothers are advised to interrupt breast feeding for 14 hours so the baby doesn't ingest radioactive milk. In addition, nursing mothers are told to avoid cuddling their babies during a 14-hour restriction period. Both these precautions are usually explained to patients in advance of their appointment and are needed to minimise the radiation dose to the baby. Very occasionally, for some scans, breast feeding must be suspended for longer periods or terminated completely. In such cases, this would be discussed with the patient in advance to allow them to plan accordingly.

Radiation protection for staff

In general, only health care staff members working in the Nuclear Medicine department are potentially at any significant risk from gamma radiation emitted from patients having diagnostic RNI examinations. Occupational exposure to Nuclear Medicine staff is carefully monitored (this is known as radiation dosimetry) and they receive specific training to ensure they perform scintigraphic examinations in a way that minimises their risk.

When patients are returning to a hospital ward after their scintigraphy examination, the nursing staff will sometimes be given special instructions. These are dependent on the type of scan the patient has had and include instructions on how to deal with the spillage of urine, faeces or vomit and the storage of waste materials and soiled linen following such accidents. In most cases however, general nursing procedures will provide adequate protection for staff on the hospital ward. If there are pregnant staff on the ward who are likely to have prolonged contact with radioactive patients, they should contact the Nuclear Medicine department for advice – each department will have its own locally agreed **protocols**.

Patient preparation and positioning

There is very little specific patient preparation for the majority of scintigraphic examinations. However, some RNI examinations such as gastric (stomach), oesophageal (food pipe), or hepato-biliary (liver and bile ducts) scintigraphy do require the patient to starve beforehand. Patients having cardiac (heart) or brain **perfusion** scintigraphy must not consume any caffeine prior to the scan, and patients having thyroid or parathyroid scintigraphy are checked to see if they are taking any medicines that might interfere with the radionuclide uptake – this would also include the recent administration of iodine based radiographic contrast agents.

Any specific preparation instructions will always be given to the patient in advance; it is important that patients read and understand the instructions they are given and let the radiographer know if they have not been able to follow them.

Patients for scintigraphy should be well **hydrated** – they should drink plenty of fluids before, during and after their RNI examination as this helps to 'wash out' the radiotracer from their body. As well as minimising the radiation dose to the patient, this also improves the quality of the images, for instance in bone or renal scintigraphy, by reducing the amount of radiopharmaceutical retained in the soft tissues.

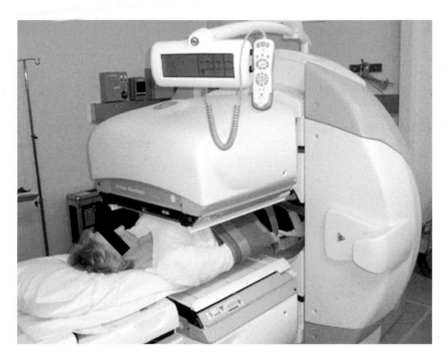

Figure 4.5 A modern dual-header gamma camera with the patient lying on the couch (pallet) between the two detector surfaces

Patient positioning against the gamma camera is different for each type of examination. Modern gamma cameras are often 'dual-headed', incorporating two detector surfaces and an intervening 'pallet', or couch, on which the patient lies (see Figure 4.5). With this arrangement the patient lies on their back (supine) on the pallet, which is then positioned between the camera heads – the camera heads are then moved as close to the patient as possible to maximise gamma radiation detection and thus obtain high quality images. If the camera heads are too far away, it has a similar 'blurring' effect to the **geometric unsharpness** described in Chapter 1 (see Figure 4.6). Sometimes the patient will have to sit or stand resting against the gamma camera – this is better for those patients who suffer from claustrophobia.

As with many other diagnostic imaging techniques, patients must be able to keep still during their nuclear medicine examination, although it is not necessary for them to hold their breath. Most individual (static) images only take a few minutes to acquire, but it is often necessary to collect a series of images while a patient is in the same position. Some of the longer dynamic studies can last up to an hour and during these the radiographer will take great care to make the patient as comfortable as possible and will also make sure they have adequate pain control. This will help patients comply with instructions to keep still and will help to produce good quality images.

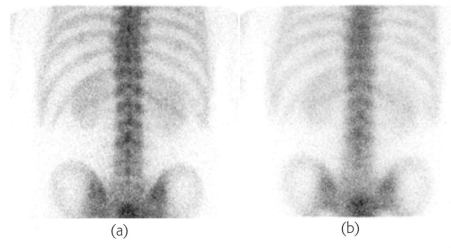

(a)   (b)

Figure 4.6 (a) Geometric unsharpness is minimised when the gamma camera is as close to the patient as possible. (b) If the patient is too far away from the gamma camera the scintillation dots appear 'blurred'

CLINICAL APPLICATIONS OF SCINTIGRAPHY

Scintigraphy is different to most other diagnostic imaging techniques as it demonstrates physiology and the distribution of organ function. Disease processes often produce a change in organ physiology much sooner than they produce a change in anatomical structure or shape – scintigraphic imaging allows these early physiological changes to be diagnosed and measured. The ability of scintigraphy to assess physiological function gives it a key role in early diagnosis, accurate disease staging and assessment of response to treatment.

Although the ability of scintigraphy to detect physiological changes early is good (that is, the examination has high **sensitivity**), scintigraphy does lack **specificity**. This means it is not always possible to tell exactly what is causing the alteration in physiology and sometimes doctors will need to refer patients with 'positive' or abnormal RNI examinations for other imaging tests for clarification.

Bone scintigraphy

Scintigraphy can be performed to look for **metastases**, **fractures**, infection and inflammation in bones – all these conditions are associated with an increased blood supply to the affected area.

For a scintigraphic examination of the **skeleton**, the patient has an intravenous injection of Tc99mHDP. The radiopharmaceutical is then distributed throughout the body by the **systemic circulation** and taken up into the bones via their blood supply. The Tc99mHDP is extracted from blood by osteoblasts (microscopic bone cells involved in bone formation, remodelling and repair) and accumulates in the bone. Any increase in the normal blood supply to the bones or alteration in the rate of bone formation or repair will cause an abnormal increase in the uptake and accumulation of the radiotracer. This means a higher number of gamma photons will be emitted from these areas; more scintillations will result in denser corresponding areas of 'dots', known as '**hot spots**', on the scintigraphic images (see Figure 4.7).

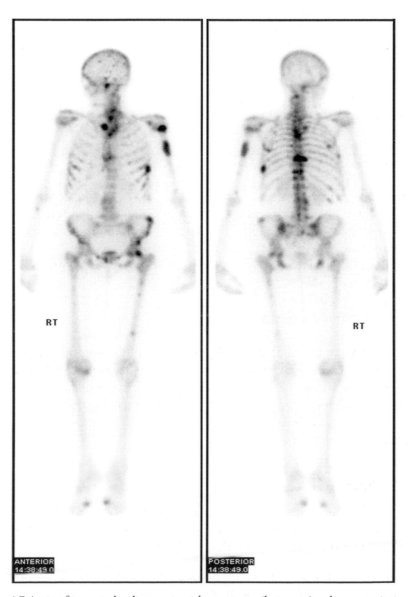

Figure 4.7 Areas of increased radiotracer uptake appear as 'hot spots' on bone scan images: this patient has multiple metastases (secondary tumours) from a primary breast cancer

Static images are routinely acquired two to three hours after the radio-nuclide injection has been given to allow enough time for the radioactivity to clear from the blood and soft tissues and accumulate in the bone – this ensures that good quality images of the skeleton can be acquired. A full bone scan lasts approximately 30 minutes. Patients are encouraged to drink plenty of fluids during the time delay to help clear radioactive material from soft tissue structures and make the bones stand out more clearly in the images. Sometimes images are acquired quite soon after the injection – in the arterial or 'blood pool' phase – to give valuable information if a recent fracture or active infection is suspected.

Lung scintigraphy

Lung scintigraphy is used mainly in the diagnosis of pulmonary embolism (PE) – blood clots in the lung. These occur, for instance, when blood clots that have formed in the legs (deep vein thrombosis – DVT) travel up the venous system of the body, pass through the heart and become trapped in the lung arteries. Initially this cuts off the blood supply (perfusion) to the area of lung supplied by the artery, but does not affect air entry (ventilation) to the corresponding lung spaces. Scintigraphy can be used to image both ventilation and perfusion – the V/Q scan (see Figure 4.8).

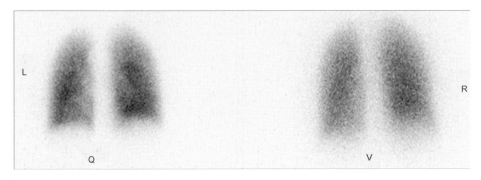

Figure 4.8 V/Q scan images: ventilation (air supply) and perfusion (blood supply) to the lungs show no evidence of pulmonary embolus (pulmonary artery blood clots)

Case study

Angela was suffering from shortness of breath and some chest pain. Dr Stevens was concerned because Angela had recently had a long airline flight from Australia and he thought she might have a blot clot on her lung. Angela was referred to the Nuclear Medicine department for a V/Q scan.

When Angela arrived for her RNI examination Sally, the radiographer, explained that she would do the ventilation images first and that she would be placing a small mask over Angela's nose and mouth and asking her to inhale (breathe in) some radioactive Krypton gas. Although this sounded a bit alarming, Sally explained that it would not affect Angela's breathing and she would feel no different. Over the next few minutes, as Angela inhaled through the mask, Sally moved Angela near to the gamma camera and asked her to keep still in a variety of standing and sitting positions so she could collect a series of static images of all the lobes and segments of Angela's lungs.

Sally then asked Angela to lie down and gave her a small injection into a vein on the front of her arm near the elbow joint, so she could obtain the perfusion (Q) images. Once again, Angela then had to stand and sit in the same sequence of positions against the gamma camera so that Sally could obtain images of lung perfusion to compare with the ventilation images.

Technical note

Lung ventilation images can be obtained following the inhalation of a small quantity of either Tc99m-DTPA given by aerosol or radioactive Krypton gas (Kr81m) inhalation through a mask. As the inhaled radiopharmaceutical fills the **respiratory tract**, and fills the air spaces within the lung, a series of static images are obtained.

Perfusion images are obtained following an intravenous injection of Tc99mMAA. Tc99mMAA, a particulate material, gets trapped in the tiny blood **capillaries** in the lung. Those capillaries that are affected by blood clots will not have any radiotracer uptake; since no gamma rays will be emitted from these areas there will be a corresponding absence of scintillation count 'dots' on the images. Unaffected lung capillaries, (namely those that have normal radiotracer uptake and thus emit gamma rays) will be demonstrated on the images.

A mismatch in the V/Q scan indicates an area potentially affected by blood clots. Pulmonary embolus is typically demonstrated on the Q (perfusion) images as wedge-shaped defects in the distribution of injected Tc99mMAA – the ventilation images not showing any defects in the distribution of inhaled radiotracer (see Figure 4.9). Although a V/Q mismatch indicates a high probability of PE, the patient must have had a recent chest radiograph to ensure that other pathology, such as **pneumothorax** (air in the pleural cavity), **pneumonia** or **chronic obstructive pulmonary disease (COPD)** is not causing the defect.

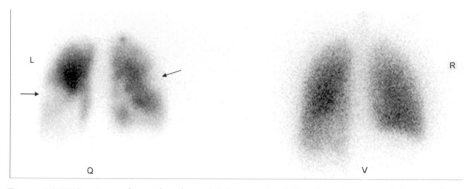

Figure 4.9 V/Q mismatch: wedge-shaped defect on the Q (perfusion) images defects with no corresponding defects in the V (ventilation) images are highly indicative of pulmonary embolus

Renal scintigraphy

Renal scintigraphy – radionuclide imaging of the urinary system (kidneys, ureters and bladder) – is most often performed when there is a suspicion that the flow of urine is obstructed. Generally, this obstruction occurs just where the ureter (the draining tube) leaves the renal pelvis (the urine collecting reservoir in the middle of the kidney) and is known as pelvi-ureteric junction (PUJ) obstruction. A renal scintigram (or renogram) is obtained by giving the patient an intravenous injection of Tc99m MAG3 and then immediately performing a dynamic study, collecting a series of rapid sequential image frames each lasting only a few seconds, for approximately 30 minutes.

The radiopharmaceutical Tc99m MAG3 is filtered from the blood stream exclusively by the kidneys and allows an assessment of the blood supply, function and excretion capability of each kidney. The renogram data can be manipulated to create images that depict renal function (see Figure 4.10) and can also be analysed to generate a time-activity curve (see Figure 4.11) and give quantitative measurements of renal perfusion, radiotracer uptake and excretion (see Figure 4.12).

SPECT: SINGLE PHOTON EMISSION COMPUTED TOMOGRAPHY

The relationship of this particular radionuclide imaging technique to conventional scintigraphy is similar to that of computed tomography – CT (see Chapter 3) – to conventional radiography (see Chapter 1). Radiation emitted in different directions from the patient is captured by rotating the gamma camera around them. The directional information is then used to create multiple scintigraphic 'slices' (see Figure 4.13). As with conventional radiography, conventional scintigraphy images give

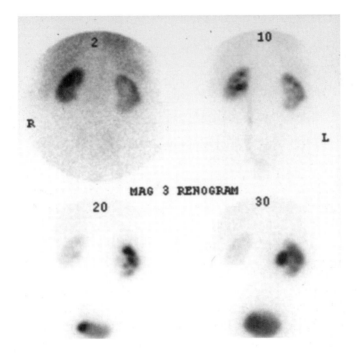

Figure 4.10 Renogram displaying renal function shows an obstruction (delayed excretion) of the left kidney

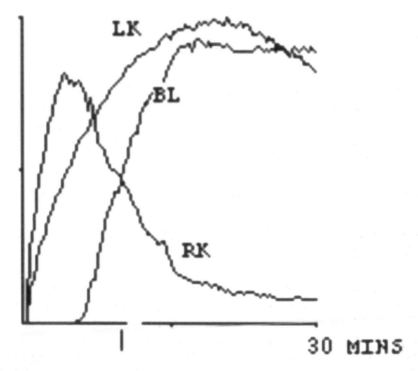

Figure 4.11 Renogram time-activity curves showing abnormally poorly draining left kidney due to an obstruction

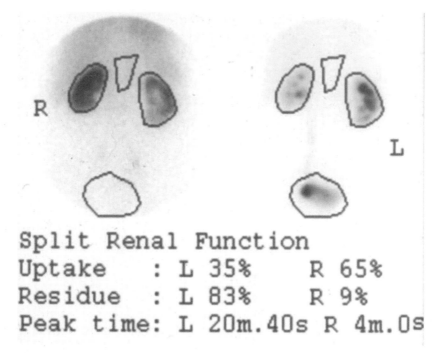

Figure 4.12 Renogram data can be analysed to give quantitative information (i.e. measurements of relative renal blood flow, radiotracer uptake and excretion) for each kidney

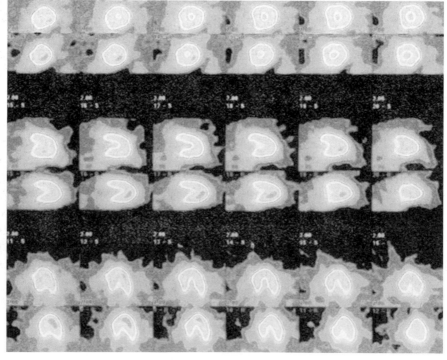

Figure 4.13 Myocardial SPECT images

only a two-dimensional representation of the body with the structures in front of or behind an area of interest superimposed. SPECT allows the three-dimensional nature of the body to be evaluated and gives the same capability for **multi-planar reformatting** as CT.

The advent of 'hybrid' gamma cameras, with combined SPECT and low resolution CT capability (SPECT-CT), has greatly improved the accuracy with which various endocrine (hormone producing) tumours, for example in the liver and parathyroid, thyroid and adrenal glands, can be diagnosed.

As a scintigraphic technique, SPECT still gives information about organ function rather than anatomy. In myocardial SPECT functional information is gained about the effects of disease on the heart muscle – the myocardium. Intravenous radiopharmaceutical injections are first given after a patient has had a period of rest, and then again after a period of supervised exercise. Comparison of the two sets of images (see Figure 4.14) can reveal areas of cardiac muscle affected by the narrowing of supplying blood vessels – coronary artery **stenosis**. Myocardial SPECT is also performed in patients who have had a **myocardial infarction**

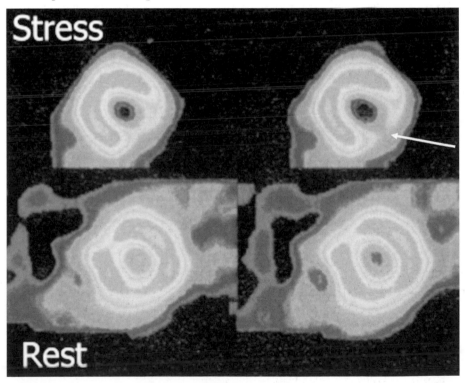

Figure 4.14 Myocardial SPECT images showing a reversible defect (arrow) in blood flow to the cardiac muscle: a perfusion defect is present during stress, with normal blood flow during resting conditions

(heart attack) to assess their suitability for coronary artery **bypass surgery**.

Bone SPECT is used to look for **occult** fractures (those that have not shown up on other imaging techniques) and for investigating complex joint pathology in the spine. Brain perfusion SPECT is increasingly being used to investigate patients suspected to be suffering from dementia, to help differentiate the cause and identify early Alzheimer's disease.

PET-CT: POSITRON EMISSION TOMOGRAPHY-COMPUTED TOMOGRAPHY

PET-CT is a recently developed innovative imaging technique that combines functional (radionuclide) and structural (CT) imaging. Essentially similar in principle to the scintigraphic examinations described earlier in the chapter, the radionuclide Fluorine-18 (F18) is labelled to a sugar based pharmaceutical – fluorodeoxyglucose (FDG) – and administered by intravenous injection. The radiotracer FDG is preferentially taken up by organs (and tumours) which have high **metabolic** demand for glucose. During radioactive decay F18 atoms emit positrons (counterparts to **electrons** that have a positive charge) not gamma rays. However, when a positron collides with an electron they annihilate and produce two gamma rays travelling in opposite directions. Detection of the two corresponding gamma rays, by a ring of detectors surrounding the patient, allows a precise determination of the location of their origin, and thus the location of abnormal cells containing the radiotracer, within the patient.

Specially designed 'hybrid' equipment allows the simultaneous acquisition of functional positron emission tomography (PET) data with high resolution CT data, and **co-registration** to produce a combined single image (see Figure 4.15a, b and c). The equipment (see Figure 4.16) looks similar to a CT scanner and, as far as the patient is concerned, the examination is very similar to having either a conventional CT or RNI examination in that they will have to lie down but be able to keep still for about 30 minutes.

PET-CT enables earlier diagnosis and staging, and thus the more precise treatment, of cancer because it is very sensitive at detecting functional change caused by abnormally multiplying cells. In addition, however, it is also very specific at determining the precise location and size of a **primary** tumour and any associated **metastases**.

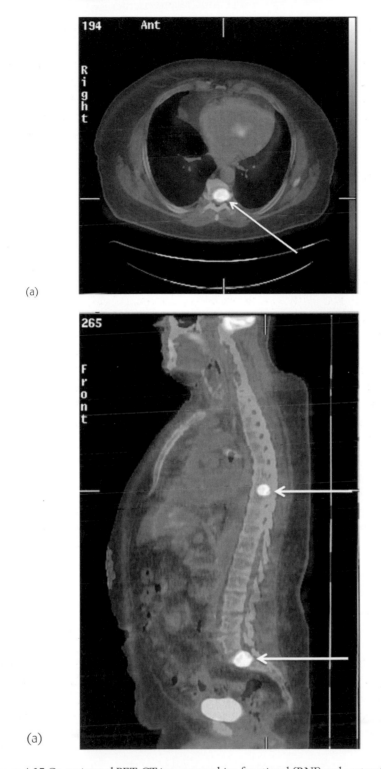

(a)

(a)

Figure 4.15 Co-registered PET-CT images combine functional (RNI) and anatomical (CT) data for precise and accurate representation of tumour size and position (arrows) in (a) axial and (b) sagittal section. (Images courtesy of Dr Andrew Scarsbrook)

95

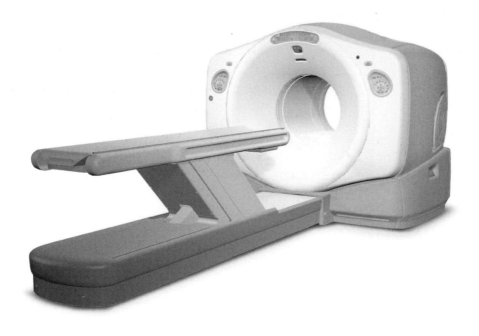

Figure 4.16 A PET-CT scanner (Illustration courtesy of GE Heathcare)

SUMMARY

Scintigraphy is a diagnostic imaging technique that primarily evaluates physiological/functional processes in the body. RNI examinations are relatively simple and straightforward from the patient's perspective, often only requiring a simple intravenous injection, and actual examination times are reasonably short. Although based on the use of radioactive substances, the associated radiation dose is relatively low; there are no significant side effects to RNI examinations and, in the majority of cases, no special precautions are necessary for patients or their families. Health care workers need to be aware of the special radiation protection measures that need to be employed if radionuclide substances or radioactive patients' body fluids are spilt accidentally.

From a technical point of view, although scintigraphy has low spatial resolution, it is cost-effective and yields functional information about the body that is not readily available using other imaging techniques.

FURTHER READING

Saha, G.B. (2006) *Physics and Radiobiology of Nuclear Medicine* (3rd Ed). New York: Springer-Verlag
This book gives more information about the physics and technology of radionuclide imaging.

Sharp, P.F., Gemmell, H.G. and Murray, A.D. (eds) (2005) *Practical Nuclear Medicine* (3rd Ed). London: Springer-Verlag
This is the best Nuclear Medicine textbook for the beginner.

Chapter 5

Medical Ultrasound Imaging
Anne-Marie Dixon

INTRODUCTION

The aim of this chapter is to increase your awareness and understanding of how medical ultrasound works and how it is commonly used. After an explanation of how ultrasound images are generated, routine clinical applications of the technique will be described to give an overview of what it involves for the person being scanned and what aspects of anatomy and pathology can usually be demonstrated during the scan.

OBTAINING THE ULTRASOUND IMAGE

Diagnostic medical ultrasound examinations are performed by a range of health care professionals including doctors, allied health professionals (radiographers and clinical scientists), nurses and midwives who have undergone specialist training and are qualified in ultrasound scanning. Most ultrasound scans in the UK are performed by specialist imaging doctors (radiologists) and radiographers. Sometimes they are also known as sonologists and sonographers to highlight their specialised skills in ultrasound scanning.

An ultrasound examination is performed by placing a small handheld device, the ultrasound probe or **transducer**, on or into the body (see Figure 5.1a and b). The transducer contains small plates of **piezoelectric** material that can generate a high frequency (ultra)sound beam. By placing the transducer in contact with the body the ultrasound beam is transmitted into the tissues and, as it travels through the body, some of the ultrasound beam is reflected back towards the body surface. A reflection or 'echo' occurs when the sound encounters an **acoustic boundary**. Acoustic boundaries exist where there is a change in **acoustic impedance**, a property determined by a tissue's density and stiffness and which determines the speed at which sound travels through it.

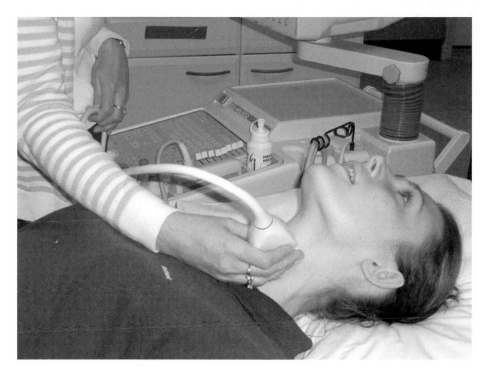

(a)

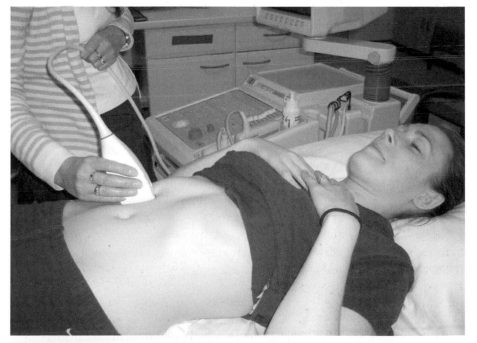

(b)

Figure 5.1 Ultrasound examinations are performed by placing small handheld transducers in contact with the body: (a) on the neck to examine the thyroid gland, or carotid arteries supplying the brain and (b) on the upper abdomen to examine the liver, gallbladder and kidney

Case study

Before Frances could have her ultrasound scan she had to uncover her tummy so that the sonographer could put some 'jelly' on it – the sonographer explained that this happens for most ultrasound examinations to ensure good transmission of the ultrasound beam between the body surface and the transducer.

Technical note

Inert **coupling gel** is used to 'equalise' the acoustic impedance differences between the transducer and the skin to minimise reflections at the body surface and ensure most of the sound is transmitted into the patient so that even the smallest echoes are detected.

At each acoustic boundary some of the ultrasound beam is reflected back towards the body surface and the transducer, and some of the beam continues further into the body to generate echoes from structures deeper. If reflected sound waves are in line with the transducer they are detected and converted into electronic signals (by the piezoelectric plates). These electronic signals are most commonly used to produce a greyscale image on a television monitor that represents the anatomical cross-section of body structures in line with the transducer (see Figure 5.2). This type of image display is known as B-mode (brightness mode) imaging, since the brightness of each pixel in the image is determined by the strength of the echo coming from the corresponding location in the patient.

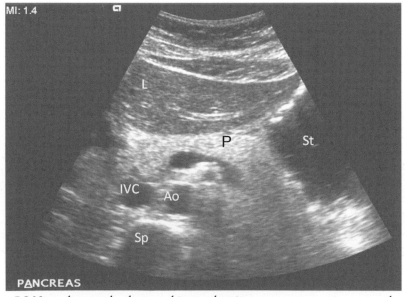

Figure 5.2 Normal greyscale ultrasound image showing a transverse section across the middle of the upper abdomen: liver (L), pancreas (P), spine (Sp), stomach (St) full of water, aorta (Ao), and inferior vena cava (IVC).

The strength of the echo depends on the relative proportion of sound reflected back from an acoustic boundary – this depends on the difference in acoustic impedance across that boundary. Large differences in acoustic impedance will result in higher proportions of sound being reflected and thus will create stronger echoes – these are displayed as lighter shades of grey (brighter) in the ultrasound image. Weaker reflections occur when the tissues are of very similar density/stiffness either side of the acoustic boundary – weak echoes are displayed as darker shades of grey in the image.

Case study

When Charlotte was having her ultrasound scan she was a bit worried to see lots of black 'holes' on the screen and she asked if this meant that there was something wrong with her . The sonographer explained that the black areas were normal 'fluid-filled structures'. She showed Charlotte her gallbladder, which was full of bile because she had been asked not to have anything to eat for six hours before her scan. Charlotte's urinary bladder in her pelvis was also 'black' in the ultrasound image – this was full of urine because Charlotte had been asked to drink a litre of water an hour before her scan. The sonographer explained that filling these structures with fluid made them easier to see.

Technical note

When there is no change in acoustic impedance as the sound travels through a structure (that is, when it is travelling through fluids such as urine, bile or amniotic fluid) no echoes are generated, so they are always displayed in black on ultrasound images. Because a large difference in acoustic impedance exists at the boundaries between soft tissue and fluid, simple cysts (filled with homogeneous serous fluid) will be readily seen when surrounded by the solid tissues of the liver, kidney or ovary.

Something to think about . . .

Can you work out why some tumours are difficult or impossible to see in ultrasound images?

It is very important that the ultrasound transducer is in close contact with a body surface and that ultrasound coupling gel is used to ensure there is no air between the transducer face and the body surface. Since there is a large difference in density/stiffness between air and soft tissue, a strong echo is generated at their interface and this is displayed as bright white in images. More importantly, as most of the sound is reflected back to the transducer, none penetrates into the body to generate echoes from further down – these areas are displayed as black in the image and are known as **acoustic shadows**.

> ## Case study
>
> Hospital patients Tom and Michael were discussing their ultrasound scans when they got back to their ward. Tom said the sonographer had found his scan quite difficult because he had been lying in bed for a few days and had lots of air in his bowel which 'cast a shadow' over the other organs in his abdomen. Michael's radiologist however had been quite pleased that he could see 'shadows' on the scan pictures because it helped him identify the small stones in Michael's kidney – this was the cause of his 'renal colic' (back pain).
>
> ## Technical note
>
> Acoustic shadows occur at interfaces of bone (or other calcified structures) or air and soft tissue or fluid. While it is a nuisance not to be able to 'see' anything in acoustic shadows caused by the ribs or by bowel gas, the effect can be used for diagnosis as shadowing is a characteristic feature of calcification, for example in stones in the gallbladder or kidney.

For ultrasound examinations performed through the anterior abdominal wall, such as general abdominal and obstetric (pregnancy) examinations, an ultrasound beam frequency of 3.5 MHz will have enough energy to reach the back of the largest abdominal organ (the liver) or the pregnant uterus (womb) in most patients. In theory, higher frequency ultrasound beams will produce better quality pictures since they have better spatial resolution. Unfortunately, however, as frequency is increased the tissue it is passing through absorbs more of the ultrasound beam's energy. In medical ultrasound, this means that higher frequency beams will not penetrate far enough into the body to generate echoes from deep structures.

Where the anatomical structures of interest are close to the surface, for example when imaging the thyroid gland in the neck or the abdominal organs of babies and small children, higher frequencies (5.0 – 7.5 MHz) can be used to get better image detail. Where structures are deep within the body, or are protected by skeletal structures such as the bones of the chest and pelvis, high frequency transducers have been adapted so they can be inserted into the body.

Case study

Mary was a bit worried when she received a letter explaining that she would probably need to have a **transvaginal** scan – where the transducer is placed a little way into the vagina (birth canal) – to look at her uterus (womb) and ovaries to try to find out why she was bleeding in between her periods. Her friend Laura told her not to worry, she had been with her father when he went for a transrectal scan (the transducer was put just inside his rectum to look at his prostate gland). Laura said her dad had found it a bit embarrassing and uncomfortable but that the staff had been very careful to ensure the room was private and that he was not in pain.

Technical notes

Intracavitary transducers can also be introduced into the oesophagus (transoesophageal) to image the heart. Some very small transducers have even been incorporated onto narrow catheters that can be inserted into blood vessels (intravascular). Intravascular transducers use frequencies around 50 MHz; this gives a very high resolution image but only of structures within a few millimetres of the transducer.

Transducer sizes and shapes will vary according to the part of the body they are to be used for. Transducers with a curved surface give a wedge-shaped **field of view** in the image – this is useful for including the whole length of organs such as the kidney and spleen or an entire cross-section of the head or abdomen of a baby in the uterus, so that accurate measurements can be made (see Figure 5.3). Large wide transducers can only be used when there is a large area free from underlying bony or air-filled structures available for scanning; smaller probes are needed when they have to be placed between the ribs or inserted into the body.

When the structures to be scanned are small and near the surface of the body, such as those in the arm, leg or neck, a transducer with a flat surface is used to get good transducer/skin contact – but this gives a much more restricted rectangular field of view (see Figure 5.4).

Case study

Before she started to scan Frances, the sonographer explained that the sound waves come out of the transducer in a narrow beam corresponding to the area of its surface and that, because only the structures in line with the transducer show up in the image, she would have to move it around and over Frances's body in order to do a thorough ultrasound

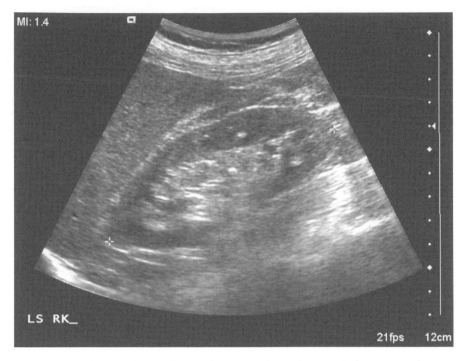

Figure 5.3 The wide field of view of a curvilinear transducer shows a whole organ, in this image the right kidney, and allows accurate measurements to be made

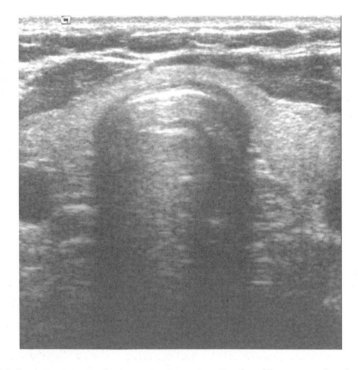

Figure 5.4 A linear array transducer gives a more restricted width, rectangular-shaped field of view: the extreme edges of the thyroid gland cannot be visualised in this image – the transducer would need to be moved to each side in turn

examination of her whole abdomen. The sonographer also explained that she would be asking Frances to move into different positions so she could get good views of her liver, kidneys, gallbladder, spleen and pancreas.

Technical note

Where bodily structures are mobile or are protected by the bony skeleton it may be necessary to use a combination of supine (lying on the back), oblique (lying halfway on the back), decubitus (lying on the side), sitting and standing positions to ensure all the organs can be seen free from overlying bone or bowel.

Something to think about...

Why do you think patients are sometimes asked to take and hold a deep breath during ultrasound scans?

Doppler ultrasound

Medical ultrasound equipment uses the **Doppler effect** to detect and display moving structures within the body.

Case study

When Albert said he was going for a 'Doppler scan' of his neck, his grandson Sam said he had learned about this in his physics lessons at school. Sam explained that you can hear the Doppler effect if you stand still and listen to a vehicle with a siren going past. As the vehicle approaches the sound of the siren increases in pitch (frequency) and as the vehicle gets further away from you the siren pitch gets lower. When Albert explained this to the radiologist doing his scan he agreed and said the transducer is like the person listening as the blood cells go whizzing past!

When an ultrasound echo comes from a moving structure (in the body this usually means from blood cells), the frequency of the echo is different to that of the original transmitted sound. Electronic software in the ultrasound machine calculates this change in frequency to get information about the direction and speed of the moving structures. The 'movement' information is displayed either by adding colour to the B-mode image pixels corresponding to the moving structures – **colour flow mapping** – or by producing a graph to show the velocity and direction of movement (vertical axis) against time (horizontal axis) – **spectral Doppler**.

Case study

At the Club one night, Albert was telling his friends about his scan to look at the major blood vessels in his neck (his carotid and vertebral arteries). His friend Frank said he'd had the same thing done on the arteries in his legs when the doctor thought he had 'peripheral vascular disease' from smoking because he kept getting cramp when he went to get his paper every morning. Another friend, Roger, had also had a Doppler scan to look at the blood vessels to his kidneys to see if narrowing (renal artery stenosis) was the cause of his high blood pressure (hypertension).

Technical note

Doppler ultrasound can be used to investigate the large vessels of the peripheral circulation (neck, arms and legs) and is also often used to demonstrate disturbances to blood flow and perfusion in solid organs that are associated with pathological conditions.

WHEN IS ULTRASOUND A USEFUL TEST?

Ultrasound is commonly used instead of, or as well as, conventional radiography early in the diagnostic pathway of patients presenting with abdominal or pelvic symptoms because it is safe, relatively quick to perform, requires minimal patient preparation and readily demonstrates most of the soft tissue organs (see Box 5.1). Ultrasound is also appropriate for imaging blood vessels as it demonstrates the arterial and venous circulations as well as the surrounding soft tissues and without the use of injected contrast agents. Ultrasound is also a good initial test when an abnormality is suspected in a soft tissue structure near the body surface since these do not show up well on conventional radiographs and other techniques, such as computed tomography (CT) and magnetic resonance imaging (MRI), are expensive, more time consuming and often more difficult to arrange.

Something to think about...

Small handheld ultrasound machines have been developed so that ultrasound examinations can be performed in a variety of clinical settings away from a central 'ultrasound department' – where might it be useful to be able to perform an ultrasound scan 'on the spot'?

Ultrasound is particularly useful for imaging children because there is no radiation hazard, there is no need for the child to stay absolutely still during the examination and parents can remain close by during the scan. Uniquely, ultrasound is the only diagnostic imaging investigation ideally suited to investigating women who are pregnant.

ADVANTAGES

- **It is safe.**
  - It does not use ionising radiation.
  - There are no known adverse biological effects in routine use, although care must be taken to ensure the recommended safety limits are not exceeded.
  - Relatives or other supporters can remain close by during the examination.

- It is relatively **quick to perform.**
  - Examination times vary from five to 30 minutes depending on the area to be examined.
  - Most hospitals have multiple ultrasound machines – with some in out-patient clinics.
  - Services can be located close to the point of care.

- It is **economical.**
  - Ultrasound machine costs vary from £5,000–£150,000 and revenue costs (per scan) are also less than CT and MRI scans.
  - One health care professional may perform, interpret and report the examination.

- It has **good patient tolerance.**
  - Most routine techniques are non-invasive with no need for injections.
  - Pelvic intracavitary examinations are associated with minimum discomfort.
  - It is painless and requires minimal preparation, although a full bladder is required for most pelvic examinations – ideally patients should fast for six hours before upper abdomen examinations.

- It has **good spatial and contrast resolution** for soft tissue structures.
  - Multiple organ systems can be demonstrated at the same time.
  - Accurate point and serial measurements can be made.

- The image is displayed in **real-time**.
  - Moving structures such as heart pulsations can be observed.
  - Needles and catheters can be monitored as they are introduced into the body.

▶

LIMITATIONS
- It is the most **operator dependent** of all imaging investigations – health care personnel performing, interpreting and reporting the examination must be appropriately trained and educated.

- **Acoustic access** may restrict the visualisation of deep structures – anatomy that lies deep and near to air-filled or bony structures is not usually demonstrated.

- The technique only allows **limited tissue characterisation**.
  - Differences between solid and fluid-filled structures are easily seen.
  - All homogeneous fluids (urine, bile, amniotic fluid, blood) look the same.
  - It is not possible to confidently discriminate between benign and malignant tumours.

- **No physiological information** is obtained, though indirect assumptions about impaired organ function may be made based on any deviation from a normal size, shape and composition.

Box 5.1 Advantages and limitations of medical ultrasound

ULTRASOUND SAFETY

Although, in theory, there is a risk of heating up tissue and bursting small gas bubbles (cavitation) within the body if the ultrasound energy used is too high, in routine clinical practice significant adverse effects from these phenomena have never been observed. It is nevertheless important that ultrasound users are adequately trained and aware of the potential hazards in order that they can operate the machines within the recommended safety limits (EFSUMB, 2006).

PREPARING FOR AN ULTRASOUND EXAMINATION

Before examinations of the upper abdomen, patients should follow a 24-hour low residue diet or fast for six hours to minimise abdominal gas and fill the gallbladder. Approximately 1–1.5 litres of water should be drunk about one hour before a **transabdominal** pelvic ultrasound examination to ensure the bladder is full during the examination. For all other ultrasound examinations, the only preparation required is to uncover the area of the body against which the transducer will be placed. When there is a risk that coupling gel might get onto clothing, examination gowns will be provided.

CLINICAL APPLICATIONS

The abdomen

Ultrasound is a good first-line imaging investigation when a patient's signs, symptoms, blood or urine tests suggest an abnormality in the upper abdomen. Patients with a clinical history of jaundice, right upper quadrant or loin pain, blood in the urine and those with a palpable mass would be appropriate referrals.

Conventional radiography will show some kidney stones and gallstones and allow the identification of a possible bowel obstruction or perforation, but ultrasound is a more sensitive and specific test for inflammation, tumour or obstruction and when the problem is thought to relate to the liver, bile ducts, gall bladder, kidneys or spleen. Ultrasound is more sensitive than radiography for identifying fluid in the abdomen (and chest) and for evaluating the major abdominal blood vessels (the inferior vena cava and abdominal aorta). However, the pancreas lies at the back of the abdomen and is difficult to assess with ultrasound, so computed tomography (CT), fluoroscopy and magnetic resonance imaging (MRI) are more appropriate for investigating pancreatic conditions.

During an ultrasound examination patients can be promptly reassured when no abnormality is detected or when a **benign** lesion such as a liver (hepatic) or kidney (renal) cyst is seen (see Figure 5.5). In patients with more complex pathology, ultrasound can be used to accurately measure the build-up of fluid in dilated bile ducts or obstructed kidneys and to measure tumours and their effect on surrounding tissues. Although, in some cases, the ultrasound features of a tumour make it more likely to be benign or make it very suspicious of **malignancy**, ultrasound appearances are not 100 per cent certain and a sample of tissue is needed. A tissue biopsy is often obtained by passing a thin needle through the skin and into the tumour. If this is done while watching the needle in real time on the ultrasound television monitor the procedure is safe and accurate.

The pelvis

Pelvic ultrasound is particularly used for looking at the urinary bladder, the internal reproductive organs in women – the uterus (womb) and ovaries – and the male prostate gland. Typical clinical indications for pelvic ultrasound will include abnormally heavy or frequent menstruation (menorrhagia), suspected ovarian cysts, blood in the urine (haematuria) and difficulty in emptying the bladder.

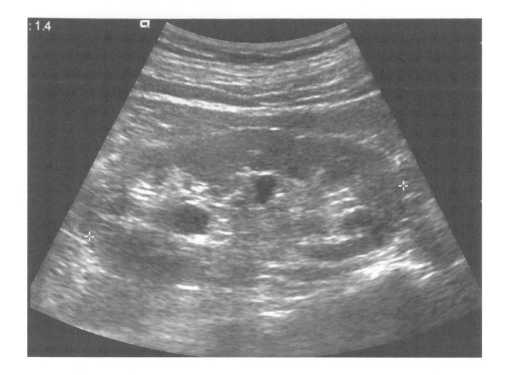

Figure 5.5 Simple cysts (there are two in this kidney) are filled with homogeneous fluid and are echo-free (black) on ultrasound images

The bladder is examined through the anterior abdominal wall and must be full of urine to demonstrate stones and tumours and to assess how well it empties when a patient goes to the toilet – men with an enlarged prostate gland typically have trouble emptying their bladder. Better images of the uterus and ovaries in women and of the actual prostate gland in men are obtained using intracavitary transducers because of their higher frequency and thus better spatial resolution.

Case study

Whenever Dr Wells is performing ultrasound examinations by putting a transducer into a patient's vagina or rectum (gynaecology or prostate ultrasound), or scanning another intimate area like, for example, a woman's chest for a breast ultrasound, he asks Sheila, the health care assistant, to come into the examination room to act as a chaperone (RCR, 1998).

Dr Wells is also careful to ask patients if they are allergic to anything before doing transvaginal and transrectal ultrasound examinations. This is because the transducers are covered in a protective sheath before they are inserted into the body; some of these covers may contain latex which can induce an allergic reaction (Bronshtein *et al.*, 1996; Fry *et al.*, 1999).

For more details on **allergies** and **chaperones**, see Chapter 9.

Benign **gynaecology** conditions such as **fibroids** are easily seen and measured (see Figure 5.6) and this information can help women and their health carers decide which method of treatment is likely to be best for them. The womb lining, the **endometrium**, can be accurately measured during a transvaginal scan and this measurement is used to help diagnose the cause of unusual vaginal bleeding (see Figure 5.7). Most often abnormal vaginal bleeding is just due to hormonal imbalances, but benign tumours (such as **polyps**), are not uncommon. Occasionally, particularly after the menopause, endometrial cancer can be the cause of abnormal bleeding and a biopsy is required to confirm this.

In women with fertility problems a series of ultrasound scans over time can show how the endometrial thickness and egg follicles in the ovaries

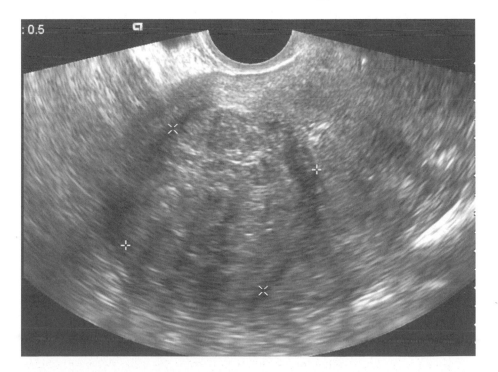

Figure 5.6 Benign fatty/muscular tumours in the uterus (fibroids) are common: this 5 cm diameter one is easily identified on a transvaginal scan as a definite round mass with a different greyscale appearance to the rest of the uterus

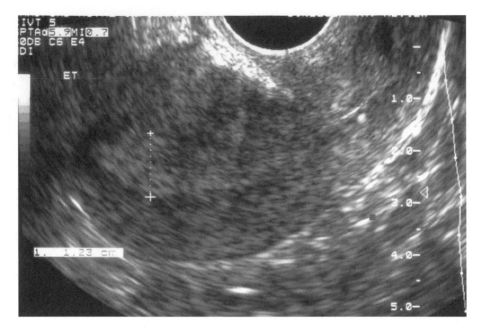

Figure 5.7 Accurate measurements of the thickness of the womb lining (the endometrium) can be made using a transvaginal ultrasound

change during the woman's menstrual cycle. This can help determine the best time to put 'test-tube babies' into the womb.

Obstetric ultrasound

Medical ultrasound has been used for over thirty years to examine babies before they are born and today all pregnant women are entitled to at least one ultrasound scan. Obstetric ultrasounds account for approximately 40 per cent of all ultrasound examinations carried out.

Pregnant women and their families often consider an ultrasound scan to be one of highlights of their antenatal care (Garcia *et al.*, 2002), but it is important to remember that the main 'clinical' purpose of ultrasound in pregnancy is to identify babies who have major problems that might not be compatible with normal independent life.

Case study

All pregnant women are offered one or two ultrasound scans when they are pregnant – this is an example of its use for 'population screening'.

When Barbara was told about her 'pregnancy scan' the midwife explained that there was a small possibility that it would show that there was something wrong with the baby. The midwife explained that it was important Barbara realised this before she agreed to have the scan.

Technical note

In any circumstances when an ultrasound examination is performed as a 'screening test' on a 'well' person, health care workers must explain the possibility and consequences of an abnormality being revealed. Only if this is done can the person really give **'informed consent'** and 'opt in' to the screening programme. Health care workers should also point out that people can 'opt out' of screening programmes if they prefer not to know about problems or would not wish to do anything about it (Whittle *et al.*, 2000).

Many people would argue that ultrasound has a beneficial psychological role even in 'normal' pregnancies and affords an exciting opportunity for 'baby bonding'.

Case study

Charlie and Laura were thrilled to see their baby's heart beating on the ultrasound scan when Laura was only six weeks pregnant and the baby, known at this stage as an embryo, was only about 4 mm long (Chudleigh and Thilaganathan, 2004, p. 39). The sonographer showed them the table she used to work out the **gestational age** – on this Charlie and Laura could see that at eight weeks pregnant their baby would still be less than 15 mm long and that at 12 weeks gestation the baby – by then known as a 'fetus' – would be fully formed and about 6 cm long (Chudleigh and Thilaganathan, 2004, p. 239).

Routine scans offered to women are usually performed about a third of the way (10–13 weeks) and half way (18–20 weeks) through a pregnancy (NICE, 2003b). At the first scan the baby is measured to determine its gestational age and to estimate when it is likely to be born. At the second scan the baby is checked in more detail to see if it has formed properly and is developing normally. Ultrasound examinations will reveal when a woman is expecting twins, triplets or even more babies (see Figure 5.8). Pregnant women who experience pain or bleeding and those who have underlying major health problems such as diabetes are usually given extra scans in a specialist (early pregnancy or fetal assessment) unit.

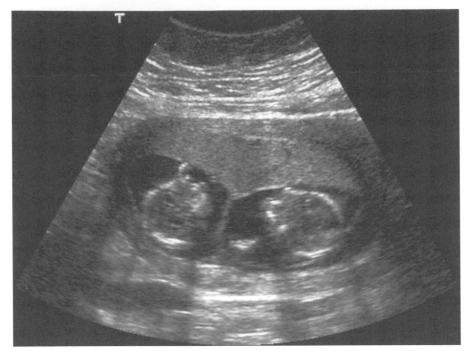

Figure 5.8 Multiple (twin or triplet) pregnancies can be detected with obstetric ultrasound – this image shows the heads of two fetuses in separate amniotic sacs

Obstetric ultrasound examinations are tailored according to the stage of pregnancy at which they are performed (see Table 5.1).

In the very early stages of pregnancy the examination is usually performed transvaginally (see Figure 5.9); later on the examinations will be performed transabdominally (see Figure 5.10).

Case study

Laura was asked to drink about a litre of water or fruit juice an hour before her 20-week ultrasound appointment time and found this quite uncomfortable – she had not had to do that for her six-week scan. Once she lay down for her scan however Laura did not feel too bad and she asked the sonographer, Angela, why she had had to drink all the water this time. Angela explained that she needed Laura to have a full bladder for a transabdominal scan (the six-week scan had been done transvaginally) in order that the baby's head was pushed out of the pelvis to allow her to measure it accurately and so she could see how close the placenta (afterbirth) was to the birth canal.

Stage of pregnancy	Clinical indications for ultrasound	Purpose of ultrasound examination
Weeks 5–12	Pain or bleeding	*Early pregnancy scan* Check that the pregnancy is in the womb and not **ectopic** Check that the baby is alive – watch for heart pulsations Identify when a miscarriage is happening
Weeks 10–13	Routine screening for Down's syndrome – offered to all women Estimate due date	*Dating scan* Measure **nuchal thickness** at back of baby's neck Measure Crown Rump Length (CRL) and calculate gestational age
Weeks 5–12	Suspected twins – excessive vomiting, previous twins or twins run in family	Count number of babies and try to see if they are 'identical' – these need closer watching as there is a higher risk of abnormality and pregnancy complications
Weeks 18–20	Routine screening – all women	*Fetal anomaly scan* Measure baby's head and leg to work out gestational age and estimate date of delivery if not done earlier Check to see if any structural abnormalities can be seen in the baby
Weeks 28–40	Mother has previously had very small babies or stillbirths Multiple pregnancies – twins, triplets, etc. Mother has a condition, e.g. diabetes, HIV, that may affect the baby's growth or well-being	*Growth scan* Measure each baby's head and abdomen and plot these on standard charts to assess the growth pattern
Week 36	Mother is losing blood or placenta was seen to cover birth canal at 18–20 week scan	*Placenta scan* Check to see if placenta is still covering birth canal – if so the doctor may recommend a Caesarean section birth
Weeks 36–42	Midwife or obstetrician suspects baby is 'upside down' – breech position	*Presentation scan* Identify if baby's head, bottom or feet are nearest the birth canal

Table 5.1 Use of ultrasound scans in pregnancy

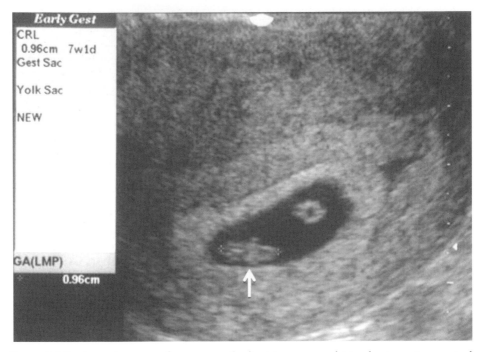

Figure 5.9 In the early stages of pregnancy the best images are obtained using a transvaginal approach – this embryo (arrow) is less than 1 cm in length (equivalent to just over seven weeks gestational age)

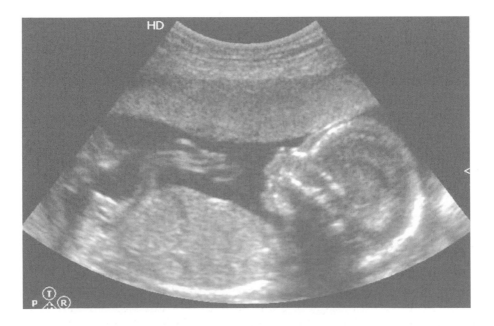

Figure 5.10 At the routine obstetric ultrasound performed between 18 and 20 weeks pregnant, a transabdominal approach is used

Additional scans are performed if a woman or her midwife or obstetrician think there might be a problem with the baby. These may be undertaken at another hospital (tertiary referral centre) where samples of the placenta (chorion villus sampling), or the fluid surrounding the baby (amniocentesis), or the baby's blood (cordocentesis) can be taken by inserting a needle into the womb and guiding it into place using the real-time ultrasound image (see Figure 5.11).

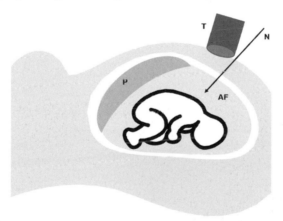

Figure 5.11 Amniocentesis: the ultrasound transducer (T) is placed on the pregnant woman's abdomen to guide a needle (N) into the amniotic fluid (AF) surrounding her baby to obtain a sample of fluid for analysis, without puncturing the placenta (P)

Superficial soft tissue structures

Soft tissue structures that lie close to the surface of the body show up very well on ultrasound images, making the test an excellent initial investigation for the thyroid gland, the breasts and the scrotum. The most common pathology in patients with a definite 'lump' to feel is a cyst – these are usually round and black on the ultrasound images and are obvious and different to solid tumours (see Figure 5.12a and b). When

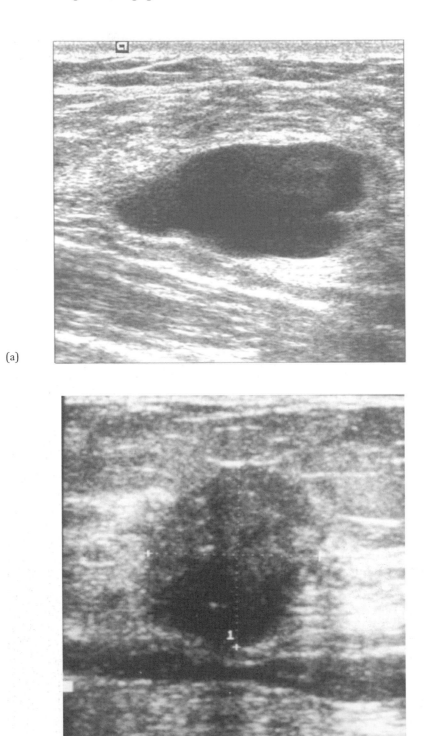

(a)

(b)

Figure 5.12 A cyst (a) and a cancerous tumour (b) in the breast have very different ultrasound appearances

solid tumours are present they can be accurately measured and, if required, needles can be guided into them to obtain a sample of tissue to check whether they are benign or malignant.

Musculo-skeletal ultrasound

Ultrasound is increasingly being used to look at the muscles, tendons and ligaments of joints (see Figure 5.13) since conventional radiographs only show the bones in detail. It is easy for the sonographer to put the transducer exactly over a point where a patient feels pain or a lump. Sometimes a patient only feels something wrong at a joint when they move it and this can be watched in 'real-time' during an ultrasound examination. Ultrasound can be used to guide needles into a joint cavity to take out excess fluid or to inject pain-relieving drugs. Ultrasound has greater spatial resolution and is quicker and cheaper to perform than MRI (see Chapter 6), but both techniques are often performed as it is easier to get reproducible (and recognisable) images showing bony, vascular and soft tissue anatomy with MRI.

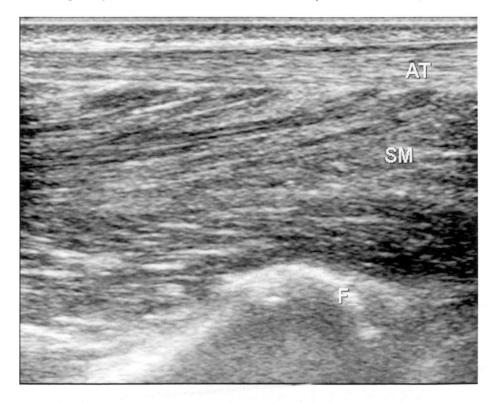

Figure 5.13 Ultrasound is good for demonstrating the muscles, tendons and ligaments at a joint: this image shows the Achilles tendon (AT), soleus muscle (SM) and the fibula, or ankle bone (F)

Vascular ultrasound

Ultrasound is a safe alternative to angiography (see Chapter 2) for looking at the blood vessels. In addition to being a radiation-free technique it allows arteries and veins to be assessed at the same time (see Figure 5.14) and it allows the structures surrounding the blood vessels to be investigated for other causes of a patient's symptoms. Vascular ultrasound is commonly used to identify arteries that are narrowed (stenosed) or blocked (occluded), particularly those supplying the legs and the brain, to check for blood clots in the veins of the leg (deep vein thrombosis – DVT) and to identify and map out vessels prior to surgical procedures such as varicose vein stripping.

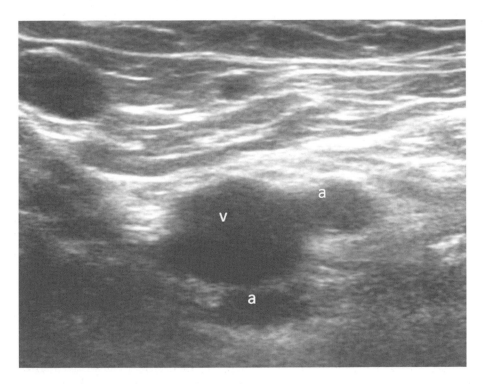

Figure 5.14 Arteries (a) and veins (v) can be seen at the same time using ultrasound imaging and no radiographic contrast agents are needed

On ordinary B-mode ultrasound images blood vessels can be seen as black (fluid filled) channels. However, when they are very narrow or very small and deep within solid organs, they can be hard to see. Doppler ultrasound can be used to fill the channel (lumen) of blood vessels with coloured pixels in the ultrasound image, making them easier to locate. Spectral Doppler is used to measure and compare the speed at which blood is flowing in vessels or in different parts of vessels. As well as directly measuring the calibre of vessels on the B-mode images, mathematical calculations can be used to work out relative diameters along a vessel from the flow velocities as fluids flow faster through narrower channels.

Case study

Frank was regularly attending hospital for ultrasound scans on his neck to check the blood flow velocities in the carotid arteries supplying his brain. He said the doctor could hear a funny vibration (a carotid bruit) when listening to his neck with a stethoscope, which meant his arteries might be getting 'furred up'. Although at Frank's first scan the vascular technician had said his arteries were only slightly narrowed, he had to go back every six months to check if they were getting worse.

Technical note

Vascular screening programmes allow doctors to monitor 'high risk' patients so that they can offer (sometimes risky) treatments at the point when the risk associated with the treatment procedure is statistically less than the risk of the blood vessel becoming blocked or rupturing.

An operation to 'clean out' the neck arteries, carotid endarterectomy, can prevent people having blackouts and strokes.

SUMMARY

When appropriately and selectively used, ultrasound is a valuable additional or alternative examination to the plain 'X-ray', particularly in the abdomen and pelvis, and is an ideal imaging investigation for soft tissue structures close to or on the body surface. Doppler ultrasound is a safe alternative to X-ray angiography that does not require needle puncture or the use of contrast agents. As a safe and radiation free investigation, ultrasound can be used as a routine first-line test so that more costly, hazardous and less readily available tests such as CT and MRI can be reserved for unusual and complex cases.

In several situations ultrasound can be considered a natural extension to the physical clinical examination. Many non-radiology specialists are undertaking the required training (RCR, 2005) and are using small clinic-based ultrasound machines to do their own scans in surgeries and consulting rooms. Ultrasound examinations require minimal, if any, preparation and are well-tolerated by patients. In experienced and trained hands ultrasound is a cost-effective, biologically safe and clinically accurate diagnostic test for a wide range of conditions.

FURTHER READING

Bates, J.A. (1999) *Abdominal ultrasound; How, Why and When?* London: Harcourt Brace

Bates, J.A. (2006) *Practical Gynaecological Ultrasound* (2nd Ed). Cambridge: Cambridge University Press

Chudleigh, T. and Thilaganathan, B. (2004) *Obstetric Ultrasound: How, Why and When?* (3rd Ed.) Edinburgh: Elsevier Churchill Livingstone

Thrush, A. and Hartshorne, T. (1999) *Peripheral Vascular Ultrasound: How, Why and When?* Edinburgh: Churchill Livingstone

Basic comprehensive introductory physics textbook

Hoskins, P.R., Thrush, A., Martin, K. and Whittingham, T.A. (2003) *Diagnostic Ultrasound: Physics and Equipment.* London: Greenwich Medical Media

Comprehensive medical ultrasound textbooks covering a wide range of clinical applications.

Meire, H., Cosgrove, D., Dewbury, K. and Farrant, P. (2000) *Clinical Ultrasound: Abdominal and General* 2nd Ed. Edinburgh: Churchill Livingstone

Sanders, R.C. (1997) *Clinical Sonography: A Practical Guide.* Philadelphia: Lippincott-Raven

Something to think about... (answers)

Why some tumours are difficult or impossible to see in ultrasound images.
If a pathological process causes only a small (or no significant) change in tissue density or compressibility, ultrasound echo signals from the tissue boundaries between normal and pathological tissue are very weak and may be below the threshold for detection and display.

Why patients are sometimes asked to take and hold a deep breath during ultrasound scans.
Taking a deep breath will fill the lungs with air, expand the ribcage and move the diaphragm lower down – pushing all the upper abdominal organs down as well. This means that the liver, spleen and kidneys are less likely to be in the acoustic shadows of the ribs and can be imaged with

the transducer placed on soft parts of the abdomen below the ribcage. If patients can hold their breath for a reasonable length of time the sonographer can move the transducer across the abdomen to get a good look at everything while the organs are stationary.

When it is useful to be able to perform an ultrasound scan 'on the spot'. The development of small and portable ultrasound machines means that ultrasound scans can now be performed away from a hospital imaging department – some general practitioners (family doctors) and specialists in private consulting rooms have their own ultrasound machines. Ultrasound scans are now often performed in hospital out-patient clinics, on the wards, and sometimes in the operating theatres. Portable ultrasound equipment can also be found in some Accident and Emergency departments and on paramedic ambulances: this helps to identify people who need an operation as soon as possible and saves patients having to wait or go to a hospital imaging department for their scan.

Chapter 6

Magnetic Resonance Imaging
Stephen Boynes

INTRODUCTION

This chapter begins by explaining the basic physical principles that underpin magnetic resonance (MR) image production and the purpose of some of the equipment used. This is followed by an explanation of the advantages and disadvantages of magnetic resonance imaging (MRI), an outline of basic MRI examination procedures and a description of some of the routine clinical applications of the technique. Last, but not least important, safety issues for patients, visitors and staff in the MRI department are considered.

PRINCIPLES OF MAGNETIC RESONANCE IMAGING

MR images of the human body are created using a strong magnet, a radio wave transmitter and receiver, a gradient magnetic field and a computer. Each of these components has a special role in MR image production.

Within the human body there are millions of atoms, the most abundant being the hydrogen atoms found in water, fat, muscle and many other bodily tissues. Over 70 per cent of the human body is made up of water molecules, which contain two hydrogen atoms and one oxygen atom (H_2O). It is the hydrogen atoms that are imaged during an MRI scan. Because they are so abundant higher quality images can be obtained compared with imaging any other atoms. Only atoms that have an 'unpaired' **proton** in the nucleus can be imaged using MRI. Hydrogen atoms are suitable for MR imaging because their nucleus contains an 'unpaired' proton – hydrogen nuclei in fact have only a single proton. Within the atomic nucleus, each (positively charged) proton spins on its own axis. In accordance with the laws of **electromagnetic induction**, a moving (spinning) electrical charge generates an associated magnetic field – thus the nucleus of a hydrogen atom can be considered as a tiny bar magnet.

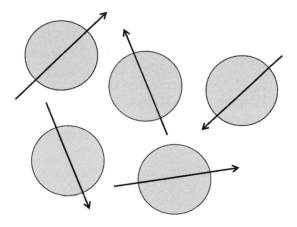

Figure 6.1 Normally the axes of spin of the hydrogen atoms in the human body are randomly aligned

Normally the axes of spin of the hydrogen nuclei in the human body are randomly orientated (see Figure 6.1). The MR scanner contains a strong magnet and when the body is placed in its magnetic field, the spin axes of the nuclei try to align themselves with the lines of force (axis) of this 'external' magnetic field (see Figure 6.2). Some nuclei align in a 'parallel' direction, and some align 'anti-parallel' – in the opposite direction. Alignment in the parallel direction requires less energy and consequently more nuclei will line up in the parallel direction and create a net **magnetic moment** (known as the 'net magnetisation vector' – NMV) aligned in the

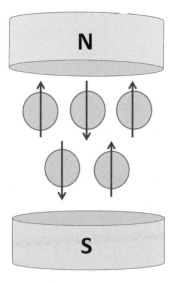

Figure 6.2 When placed within the bore of the MR magnet, the axis of the spin of the body's hydrogen nuclei aligns with its magnetic field

same direction as the external magnetic field . The magnitude (strength) of the NMV is proportional to the strength of the external magnetic field (measured in **Tesla**).

While in the strong magnetic field the hydrogen nuclei wobble, or 'precess', about the magnetic field axis (see Figure 6.3). The precessional frequency (speed of precession around the axis) is also dependent on the MR scanner magnetic field strength and can be calculated using the Larmor equation (Box 6.1).

$\omega = \gamma\, B_o$	ω	precessional frequency (Hz)
	γ	gyromagnetic ratio (a constant for a particular nucleus at 1 Tesla)
	B_o	Magnetic field strength (Tesla)

Box 6.1 The Larmor equation

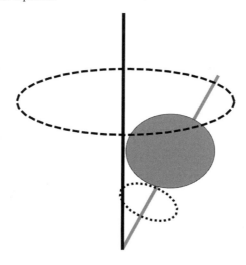

Figure 6.3 A hydrogen nucleus spinning on its axis (dotted line) and precessing (wobbling) around the axis of the main magnetic field (dashed line)

The gyromagnetic ratio is a property of the nucleus of an atom – for hydrogen it is 42.6 MHz/T (MegaHertz or 10^6 Hz / Tesla). Many clinical MR scanners have field strengths of 1 Tesla, which would thus make all the hydrogen nuclei precess at 42.6 MHz (10^6 revolutions per second).

The MR scanner incorporates a radio wave transmitter and receiver. Initially energy is transmitted into the body and can be absorbed by the hydrogen nuclei by means of a phenomenon known as 'resonance'. Resonance is the transfer of energy between two or more objects that have the same frequency. The Larmor equation is used to calculate the precessional frequency of the hydrogen nuclei at the magnet's particular field strength so that a radio wave of the same frequency can be used and a net transfer of energy to the hydrogen nuclei will occur.

Two things happen when the hydrogen nuclei gain energy. Firstly, some will gain enough energy to align in the opposite direction to the main (external) magnetic field; this reduces the strength of the net magnetisation vector. Secondly, the nuclei will start to converge on their precessional path – this creates a net magnetisation vector perpendicular (at 90 degrees) to the main magnetic field (see Figure 6.4). Thus the net magnetisation vector changes in strength and direction.

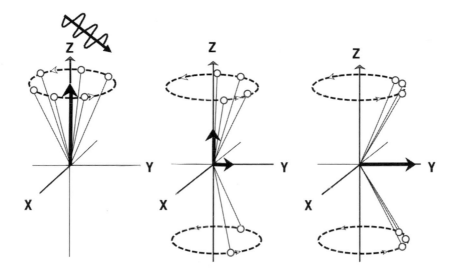

Figure 6.4 The radiofrequency pulse gives energy to the hydrogen nuclei causing them to flip into the antiparallel direction which results in a loss of the NMV in the longitudinal plane: at the same time the nuclei come together on the precesssional path and create the NMV in the transverse plane

When the radio wave is switched off, the hydrogen nuclei release the energy they have gained and revert back to their natural lower energy state. This energy is released as a radio wave that can be detected using a radio wave receiver.

Again, two things happen when the nuclei give up their energy. The net magnetisation vector in the direction of the main magnetic field recovers – this is known as 'T1 recovery' – and the nuclei start to diverge on their precessional path, resulting in a loss of the net magnetisation vector at 90 degrees to the main magnetic field – this is known as 'T2 decay'. T1 recovery and T2 decay happen at the same time but the processes are independent of each other. The T1 recovery and T2 decay processes are used to determine the appearance of the MR image, with the images being known as T1 or T2 weighted images (see Figure 6.5a and b).

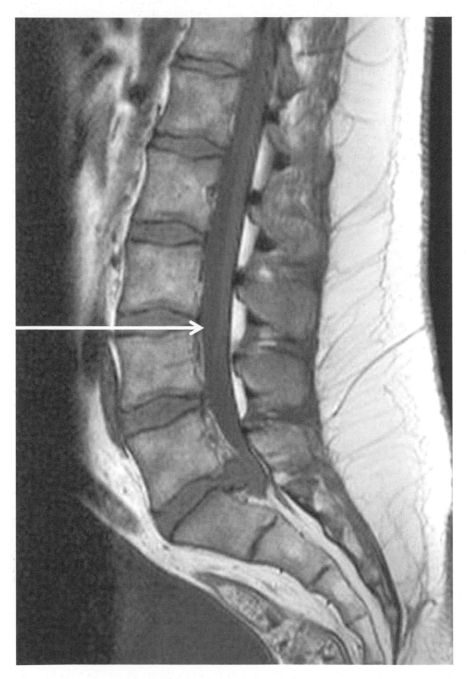

(a)

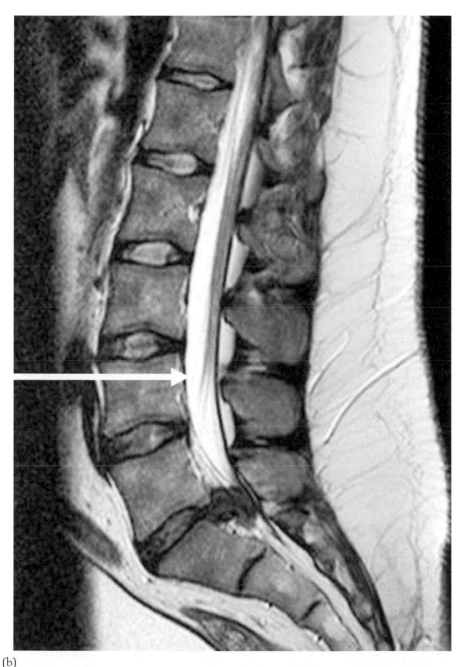

(b)

Figure 6.5(a) In this T1 weighted image, fluid (cerebrospinal fluid in the subarachnoid space around the spinal cord) appears dark on the image (arrow); (b) in this T2 weighted image the cerebrospinal fluid (arrow) appears bright on the image

In the different types of tissue in the body such as, for example, fat, muscle and ligaments, the way that the hydrogen atoms are linked with other atoms influences the rate at which they lose the energy gained from the radio wave. Because different tissues lose the energy at different rates and the different tissues have different numbers of hydrogen nuclei within them (namely, they have different proton densities) a range of T1 recovery and T2 decay values is obtained. This range is applied across a number of 'grey-scale' values in the image to provide a contrast between the different tissues by displaying them at different levels of brightness and darkness, (contrast resolution), in the image.

Equipment manufacturers make a selection of radio wave receivers designed to fit close to different parts of the body (see Figure 6.6), since image quality is best when the radio wave receiver is placed as close as possible to the area under examination. The radio wave receivers are generally referred to as radiofrequency or RF 'coils', because their basic design is that of a coil of wire.

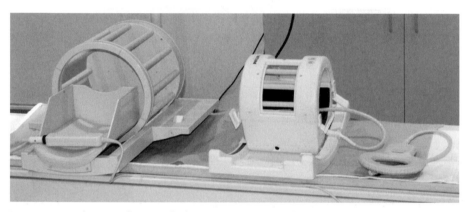

Figure 6.6 A selection of MRI radiofrequency receiver coils – from left to right: a coil for the ear, a coil for the knee and a small surface coil that could be used for a hand

So far, the energy the hydrogen nuclei absorbed has been released and detected, but to produce an anatomical picture the scanner must also be able to work out exactly where in the body the signal has come from. Three-dimensional spatial location of the emitted RF signal source is achieved using 'gradient' magnets. Gradient magnets are generated by passing electric current through coils of wire incorporated within the MR scanner **gantry (electromagnetic induction** again). The effect of the magnetic field created by the gradients is added to or subtracted from the effect of the main magnetic field, with the gradient changing the scanner's magnetic field strength in a linear fashion about an **isocentre** of the main magnet strength (see Figure 6.7a). Three gradients, one for each plane X, Y and Z, are used (see Figure 6.7b); the Z gradient alters the magnetic field strength along the long axis of the magnet, the Y gradient along the vertical axis, and the X gradient along the main magnet's transverse axis. The patient under investigation is positioned in the magnet bore with the anatomical area of interest at the magnetic field isocentre.

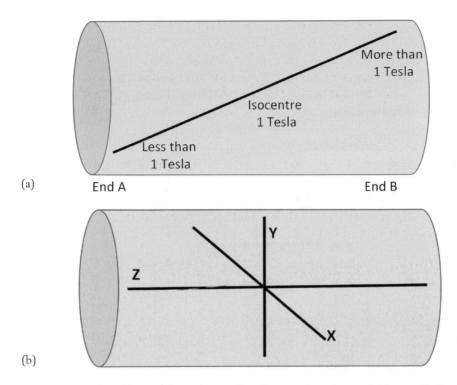

(a)

End A   End B

(b)

Figure 6.7 (a) The influence of a gradient coil in changing the magnetic field strength along the bore of the magnet; (b) orientation of the three gradient magnetic fields

Once a gradient is applied, and therefore the magnetic field strength is varied, so hydrogen nuclei in different parts of the body will precess at different rates. According to the Lamor equation, nuclei (at the isocentre) that are experiencing a field strength of 1 Tesla will precess at 42.6 MHz; those experiencing a higher field strength will precess faster and those experiencing a lower field strength will precess slower. If a radio wave of 42.6 MHz is transmitted into the patient, only the nuclei precessing at 42.6 MHz will be able to gain energy, i.e. resonate (see Figure 6.8).

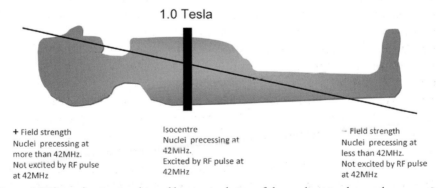

Figure 6.8 Slice selection is achieved by manipulation of the gradient to change the precessional frequency of the hydrogen nuclei

When the radio wave is switched off the nuclei that have gained energy will release it (as a radio wave) and this is detected by the RF receiver coil. As such, a radio signal has been generated from a 'thin slice' of the patient – its Z plane location is known. Once the Z plane slice location is known, the RF signal must also be located in the X and Y dimension. This is also achieved using gradients in a similar manner, with each gradient being switched on at a slightly different time.

Co-ordination of all these processes (that is, transmission of the radio wave, controlling its duration, frequency and timing, switching the gradient coils on and off, detecting RF signals from the patient, interpreting them and converting them into a suitable display format for viewing on a television monitor) requires a powerful computer. A specialist MRI radiographer operates the computer and the MRI equipment it controls from a console in a room adjacent to the MRI scanner, and from where they can also observe the patient during the examination (see Figure 6.9).

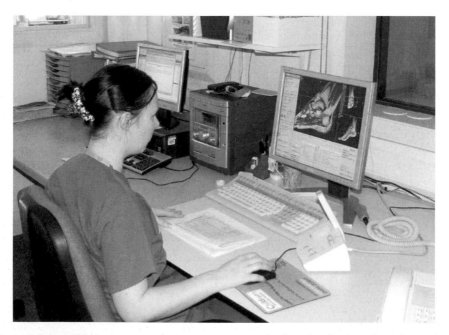

Figure 6.9 An MRI operator console – using a computer keyboard and mouse the radiographer manipulates the scan parameters; just above the mouse is the intercom for communicating with the patient

ADVANTAGES AND DISADVANTAGES OF MRI

MRI is a relatively new imaging tool that became widely available clinically in the early 1990s. Since then the number of MRI units installed in the UK and the number of examinations performed has risen annually. In 2000 it was estimated that the demand for MRI would grow between 12.5 per cent and 18.5 per cent each year (Szczepura and Clark, 2000), with this growth mainly due to the many advantages that MRI offers over other methods of imaging (see Table 6.1).

EXAMINATION TECHNIQUE

All patients should receive an in-depth explanation of what is involved in the MRI examination, preferably before they arrive in the department. For the majority of examinations the patient will be asked to lie supine (on their back) on the MR scanner couch. A variety of RF coils is available and the radiographer selects the most appropriate RF coil depending on the area of the body being examined and positions this as close as possible to the relevant anatomical structures. For example, for an examination of the lumbar (lower) spine the patient lies on the coil. Once the patient and RF coil are in position on the couch, laser lights are used to accurately position the area of anatomical interest at the centre of the magnet.

Case study

Joe had been referred for an MRI examination of his head. When he arrived for his appointment, Sally, the radiographer, checked that he knew what was going to happen and then explained that she would have to ask him a few questions so she could fill in the safety questionnaire. When this was complete, Sally asked Joe to get changed into a hospital gown and to make sure he didn't bring any magnetic objects into the scan room. Once in the room Joe was asked to lie on his back on the examination couch. When Sally had put a wedge-shaped foam pad under his knees he became more comfortable and assured her that he would be able to keep still for the scan. Sally gave Joe some ear protectors to wear and then positioned a 'cage-like' device around his head. She then gave Joe an 'emergency call button' and told him she would be watching him throughout the scan through the window of the control room. Joe knew he was alone in the magnet room and he felt it was reassuring to have control of the call button. When Sally said the scan would take about 30 minutes in total he was glad she had advised him to go to the toilet while he was waiting his turn to be scanned.

Technical note

The 'cage' placed around Joe's head is the RF coil that will receive the RF signals from inside his head. The coil is positioned as close as

ADVANTAGES	
No ionising radiation	MRI is considered a safe mechanism with no confirmed biological hazard. There are some **contraindications** to MRI scanning – see later.
Excellent soft tissue differentiation with good contrast resolution	MRI is the best diagnostic imaging technique at distinguishing between different tissue and pathology types. Unlike conventional radiography and CT where contrast resolution depends on a single physical mechanism (X-ray attenuation), the MRI can utilise a variety of physical properties to change the image contrast (T1 recovery, T2 decay, proton density).
Relatively good spatial resolution	It is possible to see structures smaller than 1 mm in MR images if the part under examination can be placed close to the RF receiver coil. Although spatial resolution is better with CT and conventional radiography, the high contrast resolution of MR compensates for this, making very small structures more conspicuous.
Multiplanar imaging capability	Computer manipulation of the gradient magnets allows the direct acquisition (as opposed to the electronic reformatting) of images in any plane. Images can even be acquired in curved planes – a technique useful for investigating the cruciate ligaments in the knee joint.
Non/minimally invasive	Most structures within the body can be demonstrated in MR images without the need for contrast agents – where used, however, they are considered safe and only require a simple intravenous injection.
LIMITATIONS	
Relatively expensive	An MRI scanner is one of the most expensive pieces of diagnostic imaging equipment to purchase and operate. Coupled with the building costs the technique is more costly per examination than general radiography, ultrasound and CT.
Long examination times	Most examinations last at least 30 minutes and patients have to lie perfectly still during this time – those in pain or who are unable to co-operate may not be able to do this. Babies and small children may require sedation or a general anaesthetic which increases the risks of the investigation. Technological developments however are reducing examination times – some images now take only seconds to acquire.
Claustrophobia	Most MR scanners are classed as 'closed' scanners, which means that they are designed like a tunnel and the patient has to lie inside – claustrophobic patients may not tolerate, for example, a brain scan where they have to lie with their head close to the magnet isocentre. Sometimes patients can be coaxed and encouraged with a sympathetic and careful explanation and sometimes the technique and/or positioning can be adapted, e.g. a patient enters the magnet feet first rather than head first. Even then 1–2 per cent of patients will not be able to proceed – patients may be asked to consent to examinations under a sedative or general anaesthetic for clinically essential examinations.
Implants/foreign bodies	Ferromagnetic materials (surgical clips, orthopaedic implants, bullet fragments) can move (migrate) within the body under the influence of the magnetic fields. This can be dangerous depending on how long they have been in the body and where they are in relation to vital organs – see later.

Table 6.1 Advantages and limitations of MRI

possible to the body part under examination to get the best signal and thus the best quality images. Patients are given ear protection equipment, and sometimes allowed to listen to music through earphones during the examination, because the gradient coils make a loud vibrating noise as they are rapidly switched on and off.

The radiographer will check that the patient's identification data have been entered into the computer before acquiring several very quick low quality 'localiser' images of the area of interest. The localisers are used to 'plan' the images that will be acquired for diagnosis. Images are planned by manipulating the various parameters that control the area of interest, contrast weighting, spatial resolution and image acquisition time. Each combination of scanning parameters is called a **pulse sequence** and each pulse sequence produces a different set of images during the examination. Each department will have its own standard examination protocols that are then customised for each individual patient. For example, where patients cannot tolerate a lengthy examination, protocols can be adapted to obtain non-standard images in a shorter time and still answer the main diagnostic question.

Case study

After Sally had done localisers and planning for Julie's lumbar (lower) spine MRI investigation, she instigated the pulse sequences to collect the diagnostic information. Julie was intrigued that the vibrating noise kept stopping and starting, sometimes lasting for three or five minutes at a time during the examination.

Technical note

The vibrating noise caused by the gradients is only heard when images are actually being acquired. It starts and stops as each new pulse sequence is carried out. For the lumbar spine, four sequences might be acquired – sagittal T1, sagittal T2, axial T1 and axial T2 – with each sequence lasting between three and five minutes.

Contrast agents

A variety of contrast agents can be used in MRI scanning, including water and pineapple juice. However, the majority are special pharmaceutical preparations containing the element gadolinium. When body tissue takes up gadolinium-based contrast agents their T1 recovery time is shortened and this gives a higher signal (brighter greyscale level) on T1 weighted images (see Figure 6.10a and b).

Gadolinium-based contrast agents are considered relatively safe and have very few adverse effects in comparison to the iodine-based contrast agents used in radiography and CT (see Chapter 2). Recent research has shown a rare but serious illness, nephrogenic systemic fibrosis, occurring in patients with **end-stage renal failure**. As a result patients with renal disease should have a blood test to check their renal function before having an MRI examination where gadolinium-based contrast agent administration might be indicated.

ROUTINE CLINICAL APPLICATIONS

With increasing technical advances and growing clinical experience the role of MRI continues to expand. The technique usually provides more information than CT about the nervous system and musculoskeletal system particularly because of its high contrast resolution and direct multiplanar imaging capability. MRI is also increasingly becoming important for imaging the vascular (blood vessel) system, breast, pelvic organs, gastrointestinal (digestive) tract and its accessory organs – the liver, bile ducts and pancreas.

The brain

MRI is the best and most versatile diagnostic technique for imaging the brain and is indicated when patients are suspected of having a **space occupying lesion** e.g. tumour (see Figure 6.11a–c). CT, however, is generally preferred for traumatic head injury, suspected intracranial haemorrhage and stroke because of its relatively lower cost, availability and examination speed.

Brain pathology is generally associated with an increase in volume of extracellular fluid in comparison to normal tissue and, as a consequence, a decrease (dark image appearance) in MR signal intensity on T1 images and an increase (bright image appearance) in signal intensity on T2 weighted images. In the normal brain a physiological 'barrier' – the blood brain barrier – effectively isolates and protects the brain. Pathological change in the brain breaks down the blood brain barrier and this allows gadolinium-based contrast agents to pass into abnormal (tumour) tissue. Thus on (gadolinium) contrast enhanced T1 weighted MR images brain tumours have increased signal intensity.

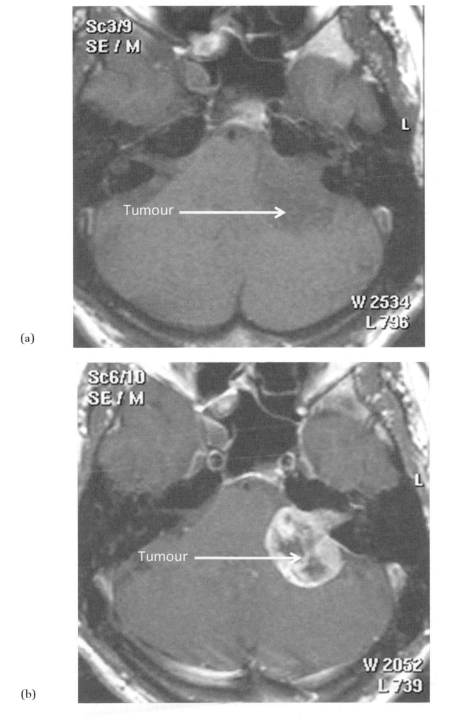

Figure 6.10 (a) A T1 weighted image of an acoustic neuroma (hearing nerve tumour) – see arrow; (b) A T1 weighted image after contrast agent administration showing a brighter signal from the tumour tissue

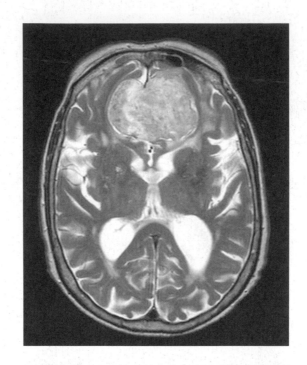

(a)

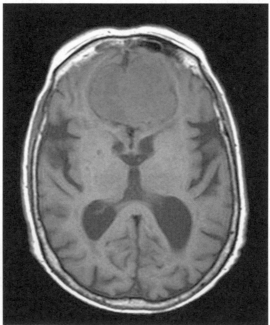

(b)

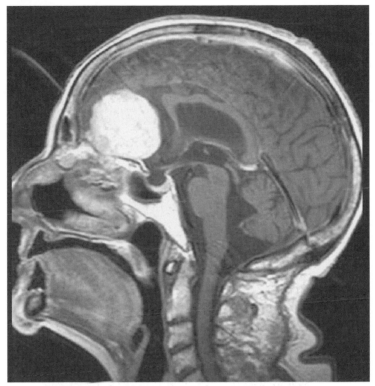

(c)

Figure 6.11 (a) T2 weighted axial image demonstrating a large well-defined hyperintense mass in the midline of the anterior cranial fossa; (b) On a T1 weighted axial image the central mass is hypo-isointense (slightly darker or same signal intensity to brain); (c) A T1 weighted sagittal image with gadolinium enhancement reduces the T1 time of the abnormal tissue and consequently shows it as a bright area

Case study

When 57-year-old Alice went to her GP, Dr Morrison, complaining of pain and numbness in her face and a sensation of fullness in her left ear, he asked how long she had been like this. Alice explained that the symptoms had come on over a period of about three months. She also told him that she felt as if she couldn't hear properly on the left side because of a ringing noise in her ear and also had been having left-sided headaches that lasted a couple of hours. Dr Morrison referred Alice to Mr Khan, an ENT (ear, nose and throat) specialist at the local hospital. Mr Khan sent Alice for an MRI scan of her internal auditory canal (inner ear).

Dr Stevens, the radiologist, diagnosed an acoustic neuroma (benign tumour on the hearing nerve) – he noted a bright mass in the T2 weighted images, a dark lesion on the T1 images and a bright mass on contrast enhanced (gadolinium) images (see Figure 6.12).

Clinical note

MRI has become the imaging modality of choice for the investigation of patients with audio-vestibular (hearing and balance) symptoms for the presence of acoustic neuroma.

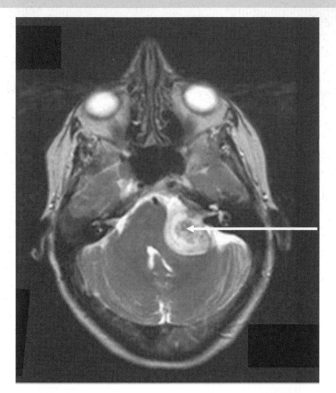

(a)

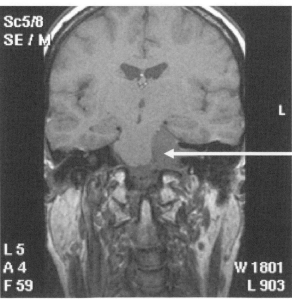

(b)

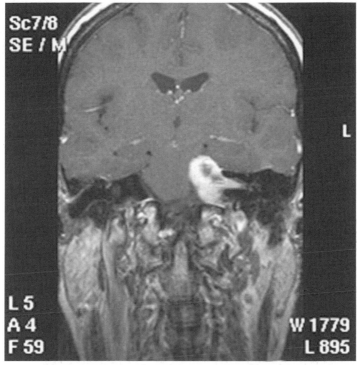

(c)

Figure 6.12 (a) A T2 weighted axial image shows a large lesion in the left cerebellopontine angle (arrow); (b) A T1 weighted coronal image with the lesion (arrow) hypo-intense (dark) compared to normal brain tissue; (c) A T1 weighted coronal image with gadolinium showing contrast enhancement along the internal auditory canal – gadolinium has reduced the T1 time of the abnormal tissue and consequently the abnormality now shows bright on a T1 weighted image

A reliable image-based differential diagnosis can often be achieved after careful consideration of the patient's demographics (age and gender), location, frequency and duration of neurological signs and symptoms (confusion, memory loss, headaches and altered function such as, for example, a personality change with, perhaps, uncharacteristic aggressive behaviour) and recognition of the characteristic imaging appearances of different tumour types.

The spine

MRI has revolutionised the imaging of spinal pathology – it is now the imaging technique of first choice. Back pain is a common and debilitating ailment, is notoriously difficult to treat, often recurring when painkillers and/or physiotherapy cease, and is responsible for prolonged periods of absence from work. Frequently, the causative injury is subtle and biomechanical rather than acutely traumatic and the resultant pathological damage is of a soft tissue (intervertebral disc/nerve root), rather than bony (spinal column), nature. Spinal MR images demonstrate bone and soft tissue structures simultaneously, allowing the visualisation of cerebrospinal fluid, bone marrow, and intervertebral discs (see Figure 6.13).

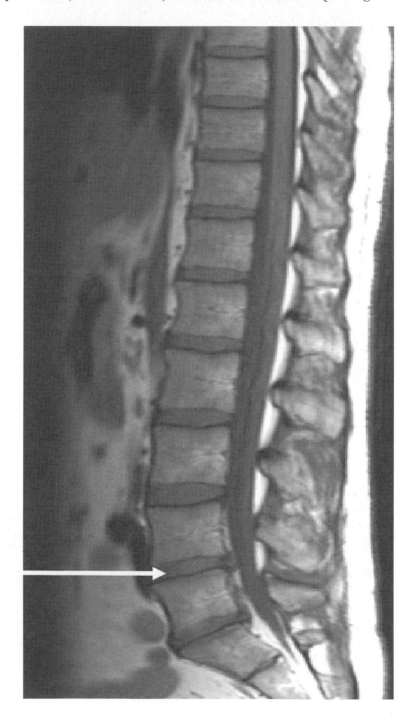

(a)

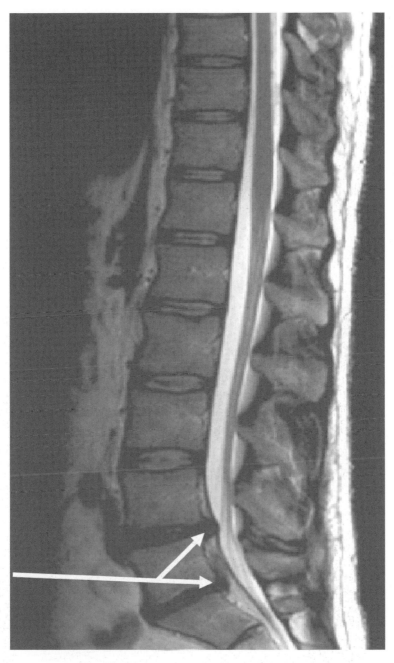

(b)

Figure 6.13 (a) A T1 weighted sagittal image: cerebrospinal fluid (CSF) has the lowest signal intensity of all spinal structures – also note the loss of disc height at L4/L5 (arrow): (b) A T2 weighted sagittal image showing posterior disc herniation (slipped disc) and loss of signal from discs at L4/5 and L5/S1 levels (arrows)

The musculoskeletal (MSK) system and superficial soft tissues

The excellent spatial resolution and good soft tissue demonstration capability of MRI make it ideal for examining joints where ligament or cartilage damage is suspected (see Figure 6.14). MRI is also very good for detecting bony fractures because the associated increase in fluid in the area changes the normal signal from bone. Many MSK injuries are often associated with sporting activities and thus with relatively young patients, so the lack of biological hazard makes MRI particularly attractive when compared with alternative imaging techniques such as CT (see Chapter 3) and RNI (see Chapter 4) that involve ionising radiation.

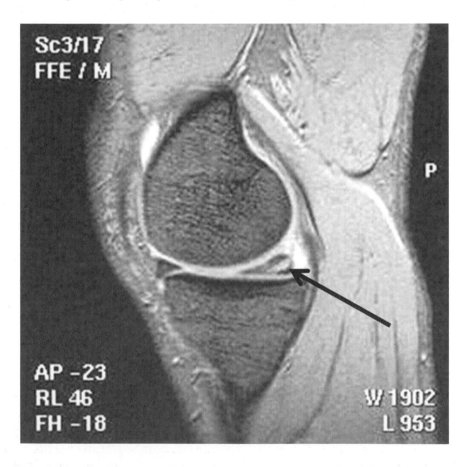

Figure 6.14 A T2 weighted sagittal image showing a tear (arrow) in the medial meniscus (knee cartilage)

MRI has become an essential tool for evaluating and staging known or potential musculoskeletal/soft tissue tumours due to its excellent soft tissue contrast and its multiplanar capability. Although tumour cell type cannot be specified from MR examinations, the use of various pulse sequences and different image weighting parameters enables some tissue characterisation. MRI can identify the tissue from which a suspected tumour arises, assess the blood supply within an abnormal mass and assess the effect of the mass on other structures close by.

The vascular system

MRI techniques can be employed to examine the blood vessels without the use of contrast agents. 'Time-of-Flight' magnetic resonance angiography (MRA) utilises the fact that moving structures (flowing blood) give a different RF signal to stationary structures. This produces detailed images of blood vessels in a non-invasive manner. However, diagnostic accuracy can be improved using gadolinium contrast agent. Contrast enhanced MRA (see Figure 6.15a and b) using a simple intravenous injection is much less invasive than conventional X-ray based angiography (see Chapter 2).

The pelvic organs

MRI is excellent for looking at the soft tissue organs (uterus, ovaries or prostate gland) and surrounding structures in the pelvis because of its high contrast resolution. Degradation of images by respiratory movement (breathing) or peristalsis (movement of the intestines) is generally not a problem in the pelvis; although anti-spasmodic drugs and/or a laxative bowel preparation are occasionally necessary. MRI is particularly useful for staging rectal (back passage) and cervical (lower female reproductive tract) tumours as it clearly demonstrates the extent of local tumour invasion and spread to adjacent supporting tissue or regional lymph nodes – such information can help surgeons decide which treatment option is best for the patient.

The gastrointestinal tract and its accessory organs

Although ultrasound is usually used as the first-line imaging test to investigate the soft tissue organs of the upper abdomen, MRI gives excellent images of the liver, biliary tree and pancreas. Patients with jaundice might be selectively referred for MRI when ultrasound has demonstrated an abnormally dilated (widened) bile duct but has not revealed the cause. MRI visualisation of the common bile duct and head of the pancreas is not obscured by overlying bowel gas as it often is during ultrasound examinations, making it more reliable for demonstrating stones which might be blocking the lower end of the duct (see Figure 6.16).

A recent development, MR enteroclysis, where the bowel is filled with contrast agent via a **naso-gastric tube**, can be used to examine the small intestine. For patients with chronic conditions such as inflammatory bowel disease, the ability to perform repeat MR investigations avoids having to utilise serial small bowel enemas using ionising radiation and fluoroscopy.

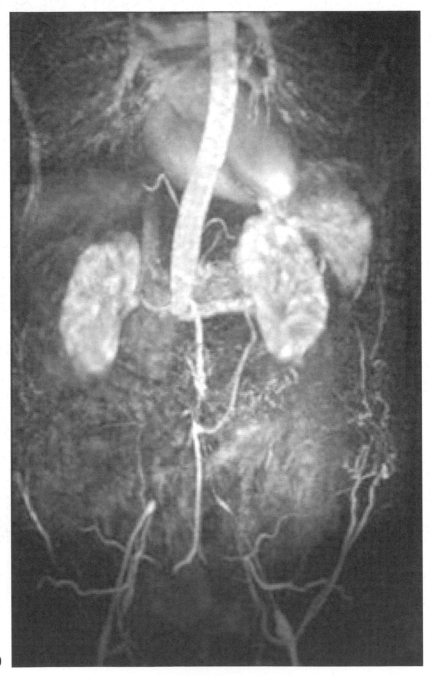

(a)

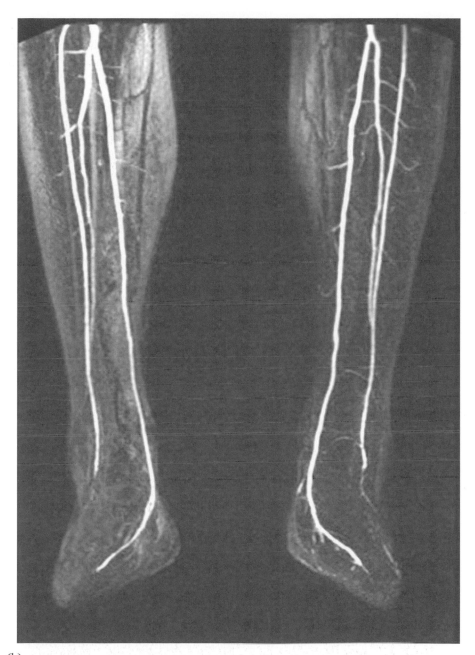

(b)

Figure 6.15 (a) A magnetic resonance angiogram (MRA) image demonstrating occlusion (blockage) of the aorta (main artery in the body) below the kidneys; (b) Blood flow to the lower legs and feet is maintained by collateral flow from vessels that bypass the blockage and arise from the arteries supplying the bowel

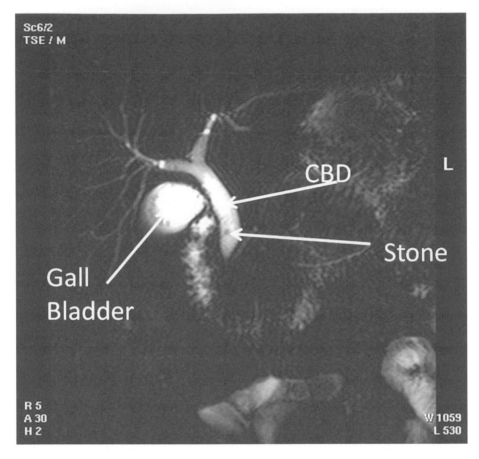

Figure 6.16 Common bile duct (CBD) stone (dark circle) in a patient with jaundice and abdominal pain; despite duct widening no stone was seen during an ultrasound examination

Case study

Melissa had been admitted to hospital with jaundice and abdominal pain and had recently been to the imaging department for an ultrasound examination. When Miss Young, the general surgeon came onto the ward later that day he explained that the sonographer had seen lots of small gallstones and had also noticed that Melissa's common bile duct (CBD) was dilated (widened). Unfortunately, because Melissa had been in a lot of pain and had swallowed lots of air, the lower end of her bile duct had been obscured by bowel gas. Miss Young told Melissa that she was going to send her for an MR scan because she thought there might be a stone in the bile duct itself and she wanted to check this before she performed 'keyhole' surgery.

The breast

MRI is not a routine examination for breast imaging but it can be used to solve problems when mammography (X-ray) and ultrasound appearances are inconclusive. Breast MRI is particularly useful for differentiating cancer recurrence from surgical scarring and for looking for leakage or rupture of breast implants.

SAFETY ISSUES

To date, no long-term adverse biological effects have been associated with clinically indicated MR imaging. However, there are a number of potential hazards associated with magnetic and radiofrequency fields which patients, visitors and health care staff need to be aware of.

The magnetic field of the main magnet extends beyond the scanner itself. The stray magnetic field, called the fringe field, is not confined by conventional building materials and so may extend beyond the walls, floor and ceiling of the scanner room. When manufacturers install the magnet they usually install 'shielding' to limit the extent of the fringe field to the scanner room, but sometimes this is not possible. Any area where the magnetic field is above 5 Gauss (1 Tesla = 10,000 Gauss), the recommended safe limit for the general public, is designated a **controlled area**.

Any patient or visitor (including accompanying health carers) attending the MRI department has to complete a 'safety questionnaire' to ensure that they do not enter the controlled area if it might be unsafe for them to do so. If a patient cannot answer the safety questions themselves, for example if they are unconscious, radiographers will study their case notes or ask close relatives for information.

Access into the controlled area is only allowed for people who have undergone **safety screening** and are under the direction of an **authorised person** – usually the radiographer who will perform the examination. MRI departments generally have locked doors that only authorised personnel can open.

Hazards associated with the main magnetic field

Dangers associated with the main magnetic field are always present because most MRI scanner magnets stay 'on' all the time, i.e. the associated magnetic field is present even when the staff are not in the department such as, for example, in the middle of the night.

Projectile effect

Ferromagnetic metals will be attracted towards the centre of the main magnet, often with considerable force, and should not be taken into the MR scanner room. Care should be taken to avoid inadvertently bringing in coins, scissors, paper clips, paging devices, stethoscopes, wheelchairs, trolleys and oxygen cylinders. Unfortunately there are reports of such instances and, in some cases, fatalities have occurred. The increase in force of attraction as you get closer to the magnet is not uniform – it is possible to move from an area of hardly any force to a point of very strong attraction in just a short distance. MRI compatible wheelchairs and trolleys can be used to bring patients from the ward to the MRI department to avoid the inconvenience of transferring patients who have been transported using traditional wheelchairs or trolleys.

Case study

After Tom had filled in the MRI safety questionnaire, he was asked to go for an X-ray examination of his eyes to make sure there were no tiny fragments of metal in them. The radiographer explained that this was routine practice for people who had worked with grinding or milling machines.

Technical note

The safety screening questionnaire should identify people who may have ferromagnetic objects in their body – this includes those with pacemakers, metallic foreign bodies, piercings, intravascular coils, filters and stents (see Chapter 2), aneurysm clips and prosthetic heart valves or joint replacements. The potential risk is that the force of attraction created by the main magnetic field will cause the ferromagnetic material to move in the body. Sometimes manufacturers will have stated that devices are MRI compatible and safe, and, in some cases, this might be conditional upon the strength of the magnetic field. A device may be MR compatible at 1.5 Tesla but not at 3 Tesla. The likelihood of movement, and resulting biological harm, can be influenced by how long an implant has been in place. Most orthopaedic implants such as, for example, joint replacements and fracture fixation screws or nails, are considered safe if they have been in place for more than three months.

The magnetic field can also potentially interfere with the operation of electronic devices such as pacemakers and cochlear (hearing) implants, so people with pacemakers will generally not be able to have MRI because of the potential catastrophic effect of pacemaker malfunction.

Biological effects

No harmful biological effects have been demonstrated at the field strengths commonly used in clinical MRI, although at high field strengths (above 2 Tesla) reversible effects such as fatigue, headache, low blood pressure and irritability have all been observed (Westbrook *et al.*, 2005). As field strengths rise with modern technological developments it will be important to assess any possible associated adverse effects.

Although there are a number of mechanisms that could potentially cause harm to unborn babies, particularly in the first 12 weeks of a pregnancy when cells are dividing rapidly, no harmful effects have been demonstrated in clinical practice. Caution, however, is still advised and obstetric use is primarily confined to the further evaluation of abnormalities that have been diagnosed during routine prenatal ultrasound screening examinations. Pregnant staff may opt not to enter the controlled area during the first 12 weeks of their pregnancy and, throughout pregnancy, they should not be present in the examination room during image acquisition (MHRA, 2007)

Hazards associated with the gradient magnetic fields

In addition to a very loud vibrating noise (see earlier), the rapid switching on and off of the gradient magnetic fields has the potential to induce an electric current in materials within the field that conduct electricity (following Faraday's law of electromagnetic induction). Certain tissues in the human body, for example nerves, blood vessels and muscle, can behave like electrical conductors, so electrical stimulation of such tissues can induce effects such as perceived flashing lights (visual nerve stimulation), muscle twitching and atrial fibrillation (unco-ordinated heart contractions due to heart muscle stimulation). Once the gradients are switched off, the stimulus is removed and these effects will stop.

Hazards associated with radiofrequency fields

Energy from the radiofrequency (RF) pulse is absorbed by the body and will cause a rise in the temperature of the tissues. The temperature rise is such that many patients can actually feel the warming effect and this is of potential concern in pregnant patients, tiny babies and in those patients with high blood pressure. MRI equipment is interlocked to prevent the radiographer selecting scanning parameters that would cause a rise in core body temperature greater than 1°C – the radiographer must program the patient's weight into the computer to allow for such calculations.

The RF antennae effect

The RF antennae effect can cause significant burns to a patient's skin due to electrical currents being induced in conductive loops. The radiographer must ensure that equipment that might cause conductive loops (for example, ECG leads and the wires for the MRI surface coils) are not left in a loop on the patient and that they are well insulated. Skin surfaces and limbs can also form a conductive loop and this is why, for instance, a patient's thighs are separated and insulating material might be placed between them.

Finally it is worth mentioning that make-up and tattoos will sometimes have a high iron oxide content and may cause burning. Patients will be instructed to remove make-up and those with tattoos will be advised to tell the radiographer immediately if they feel any localised discomfort.

SUMMARY

MRI has revolutionised medical imaging in recent years. Without the associated adverse effects of ionising radiation, the technique gives excellent spatial and contrast resolution for a variety of body tissues. Although its high cost and limited availability preclude its widespread use as a routine first-line diagnostic imaging test, it is a reliable problem-solving tool in complex cases and is emerging as the definitive single test for selected groups of patients.

FURTHER READING

McRobbie, D.W., Moore, E.A., Graves, M.J. and Prince, M.R. (2006) *MRI Picture to Proton* (2nd Ed). Cambridge: Cambridge University Press For those who would like to further explore MRI this is an affordable book that covers the basics of MR practice and theory, progressing from basic information like 'the patient's journey' and 'a week in the life of an MR radiographer', through to specialist topics and new developments in MRI.

Chapter 7

Balancing Risk and Benefit in Medical Radiology
Andy Scally

HISTORICAL BACKGROUND

Ionising radiation, in the form of X-rays, has been used to produce images of the human body since very shortly after they were discovered by Wilhelm Roentgen in 1895 (Meinhold and Taschner, 1995). The potentially hazardous nature of X-rays, and of other forms of **ionising radiation** such as those produced as a result of **radioactive decay** (discovered by Henri Becquerel in 1896), was recognised early. The first reports of adverse effects to the skin of X-ray researchers appeared in 1896 and, in 1902, the first cases of radiation-induced skin cancer were reported. In 1906 Bergonié and Tribondeau identified the relationship between the relative **radiosensitivity** of biological tissue and its **metabolic** state. They demonstrated that young cells, immature cells, highly active cells and those undergoing rapid **replication** are all more susceptible to radiation damage than older cells, mature cells and cells with low levels of activity and replication (Bolus, 2001).

Radiation protection standards were first developed around this time and they have been refined periodically since then, in light of the emerging evidence of the potentially harmful effects of ionising radiation. This evidence has been obtained through experimentation on animals, humans and cell cultures and, most importantly, from observational studies of groups of people exposed to ionising radiation. In 1928 the International Commission on Radiological Protection (ICRP) was formed and their recommendations continue to inform the development of radiation protection practices and legislation throughout the world. The most recent ICRP recommendations were published in 2007 (ICRP, 2007).

PRINCIPLES OF RADIOLOGICAL PROTECTION

The ICRP defines three fundamental principles of radiological protection. In the hospital environment these principles apply separately to patients, staff and members of the public who might be exposed to radiation. The three principles are:

- Justification – is it worth doing?
- Optimisation – what is the best way to do it?
- Limitation – how much **dose** to any one individual is too much?

Justification

In simple terms, the principle of justification requires that any radiation exposure to an individual or group of people should produce an overall benefit. In other words, if the total benefits (real and potential) are weighed up against the total costs (which include the risks associated with radiation exposure), the benefits must win.

Optimisation

For any given radiation exposure situation, if the principle of justification is met, then the optimisation principle comes into play. The optimisation principle requires that all doses, and the risks associated with doses, should be kept as **low as reasonably practicable (ALARP)**, taking into account economic and social factors. With this principle there is clearly significant scope for subjective judgement, both in considering what is 'reasonable' and how much importance should be given to 'economic and social factors'.

Limitation

The purpose of the third principle, limitation, is to ensure that no one person is put at risk beyond a certain tolerable level, irrespective of what the wider benefits to society might be. The dose level considered 'tolerable' is also somewhat arbitrary as it is determined both by the scientific evidence of the harmful effects of radiation and by social conventions as to what level of risk is considered acceptable.

One important distinction to make here is that while the principles of justification and optimisation apply to all situations, the principle of limitation applies to occupational (health care worker) exposure and to the exposure of members of the general public but does not apply to the medical exposure of patients. The reason for this is that every radiation exposure of a patient must be individually justified and optimised and the decision as to whether the exposure is justified necessarily takes into account the dose that the patient is likely to receive (see later).

CURRENT UK LEGISLATION

Several items of legislation apply specifically to the use of ionising radiation. Three items of particular relevance to medical exposures are mentioned here, although there are other important legislation requirements relating to:

- the use and transport of radioactive materials;
- workers potentially exposed to moderately high levels of radiation (Classified Radiation Workers);
- the use of personal protective equipment;
- the management of health and safety at work.

The Ionising Radiations Regulations (IRR, 1999)

The IRR 1999 outline a framework for ensuring that employees, members of the public and (to a limited degree) patients are adequately protected. These regulations govern all aspects of the organisation of radiation protection measures in the hospital environment and in other settings, and cover such things as equipment controls, that limit radiation exposure, undertaking risk assessments, marking out areas where radiation is present, control of access to these areas, dose limits, dose monitoring and the notification of adverse incidents and accidents to the Health and Safety Executive. More practical advice for employers and staff involved in radiation protection is provided in the Health and Safety Executive's accompanying *Approved Code of Practice* (HSE, 1999).

The Justification of Practices Involving Ionising Radiation Regulation SI2004 No. 1769

Some common practices that involve the use of ionising radiation have been given prior government approval and recognised medical uses of ionising radiation come into this category (see Table 7.1). The regulations cover the established uses and anyone proposing a new application of ionising radiation would need to demonstrate that it met the requirements of this legislation in order that the justification for the proposed use could be assessed (DEFRA, 2008).

Case study

Suzy, the radiographer, was checking request cards to **justify** the exposures for the people in the waiting room. She justified three requests for chest X-rays. Albert Smith was short of breath and had a high temperature – the doctors were not sure if Albert had **pneumonia** or a collapsed

---

Purpose	Classes or Types of Practice	Lead Department
5. Production of radioisotopes	Manufacture of **radioisotopes** using nuclear reactors and accelerators	Department for Business, Enterprise & Regulatory Reform
6. Production of radioactive products	Manufacture of radioactive sources, substances and **radiopharmaceuticals**	Department for Business, Enterprise & Regulatory Reform
9. Radiation processing of products	Use of gamma or electron beam radiation sources to reduce bacterial levels, sterilise, disinfect or modify materials	Department for Business, Enterprise & Regulatory Reform
16. Security screening	Use of X-rays to radiograph suspected smugglers	Home Office / HM Revenue & Customs
	Use of X-rays or gamma rays to detect people seeking illegal entry to the UK in vehicles or freight	Home Office / Department for Transport
18. Radioactive tracers	Use of radioactive tracers for medical or biological techniques	Department of Health
19. Diagnosis – medical	Use of ionising radiation in radiography, fluoroscopy, computed tomography, in-vivo nuclear medicine and in-vitro nuclear medicine	Department of Health
20. Treatment – medical	Use of ionising radiation in interventional radiology; in-vivo nuclear medicine; teletherapy; brachytherapy; radiography (for planning purposes); fluoroscopy (for planning purposes); computed tomography (for planning purposes)	Department of Health
21. Occupational Health screening	Use of ionising radiation in radiography and in-vivo nuclear medicine.	Department of Health
22. Health screening	Use of ionising radiation in radiography and in-vivo nuclear medicine	Department of Health
23. Medical and biomedical research	Use of ionising radiation in radiography; fluoroscopy; interventional radiography; computed tomography; in-vivo nuclear medicine; in-vitro nuclear medicine; teletherapy; brachytherapy and neutron activation analysis	Department of Health
24. Medico-legal procedures	Use of ionising radiation in radiography; fluoroscopy; interventional radiography; computed tomography and in-vivo nuclear medicine	Department of Health
25. Diagnosis and therapy – veterinary	Use of ionising radiation in radiography; fluoroscopy; computed tomography; in-vivo nuclear medicine; in-vitro nuclear medicine; teletherapy and brachytherapy	Department of the Environment, Food and Rural Affairs
26. Teaching, including FE and HE, and training	Use of radioactive sources, substances and radiation generators	Department for Children, Schools and Families
29. Transport of radioactive material	Transport of radioactive material by air, road, rail	Department for Transport

Table 7.1 Practices involving the use of ionising radiation in a health care setting that have received prior approval (DEFRA, 2008)

lung, so did not know what treatment would be best. Omar Hussein was a volunteer participant in an approved research study and the research team needed to know that he had no chest disease before accepting him onto the new drug trial. Maria Rodriguez had just qualified as a nurse and needed occupational health clearance before she could start her new job on a children's ward. Stefan Wozinski was waiting for a chest X-ray before undergoing a hernia repair. Suzy went to check if Stefan had any particular history that put him at increased risk from the anaesthetic. As there didn't seem to be any specific problem Suzy couldn't justify the **pre-op chest** request and went to discuss this with Stefan's consultant.

Technical note

Although the general practices outlined in Table 7.1 do not require repeated justification, it is still true that each and every medical exposure of an individual requires its own unique justification decision, made in the context of that particular individual's medical condition or other status.

The Ionising Radiation (Medical Exposure) Regulations [IR(ME)R] 2000

IR(ME)R 2000 is primarily concerned with the justification of medical exposures at the level of the individual and the optimisation of such exposures. It identifies five distinct 'roles' for health care workers and the procedures necessary to ensure that every individual medical exposures is justified and optimised. Each of the five roles identified in the legislation has very specific (legal) responsibilities (see Table 7.2).

IR(ME)R role	Responsibilities
Employer	Ensuring appropriate and adequate policies and procedures are produced and implemented.
Referrer	Permitted by employer to request a radiological procedure. Must provide adequate and correct information regarding: • the demographic details of the patient; • clinical details explaining the reasons for the radiological request.
Practitioner	Makes the judgement as to whether or not a request for a radiological investigation is justified.
Operator	Optimises an imaging procedure, jointly with the practitioner. Responsible for all other practical aspects of the exposure.
Medical Physics Expert	Provides specialist advice, particularly relating to optimisation and patient dose assessment.

Table 7.2 IR(ME)R 2000 roles and responsibilities

157

OPTIMISATION OF STAFF AND PATIENT DOSE

In practice, the process of optimisation requires the consideration of a wide range of factors. Staff doses are kept as low as reasonably practicable by ensuring that diagnostic imaging equipment and the environment are designed with radiation protection specifically in mind, through engineering controls on the equipment, the adoption of safe working practices and by using personal protective clothing and accessory equipment such as lead rubber aprons, gloves, thyroid shields and lead glass screens (see Figure 7.1a and b).

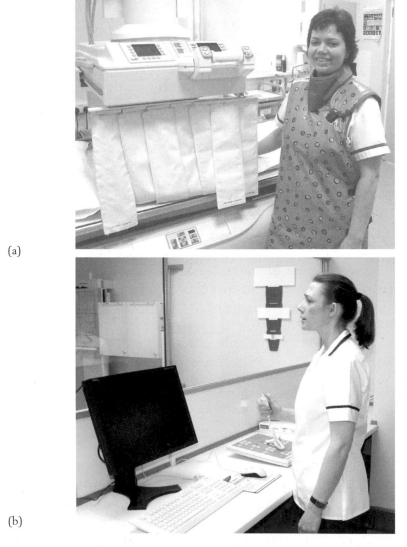

(a)

(b)

Figure 7.1 Personal protective clothing and accessory equipment such as (a) lead rubber aprons and thyroid shields and (b) lead glass screens are used to keep the staff radiation dose to a minimum

Whenever possible, health care staff will leave the room or stand behind a lead glass screen during actual exposures. Whenever staff, or members of the public such as parents and other relatives, have to remain in the room to help perform the procedure or help patients keep still in the correct position, a record of their names and the exposure details is kept.

Patient doses are optimised through the selection of the minimum number of **projections/exposures** necessary to satisfy the diagnostic (or therapeutic) requirements of the examination, by selection of appropriate imaging equipment and **exposure parameters** (factors affecting the amount and energy of radiation entering the patient) for the requested procedure, and through the use of ancillary equipment such as compression devices and the lead rubber shielding of radiosensitive tissues (see Figure 7.2).

Dose quantities used in radiation protection

The term **radiation dose** is used to quantify the risks from ionising radiation – this is a measurable quantity that is characteristic of radiation that correlates reasonably strongly with the actual risks incurred by exposed individuals. There are several slightly different radiation dose quantities, but the key characteristic of all dose quantities is that the fundamental process that they measure is the transfer of energy from the radiation itself to the biological tissue of the subject who is exposed. It is this energy transfer process that ultimately gives rise to the various hazardous effects, or potential effects, resulting from radiation exposure (see page 163). The most commonly encountered dose quantities are absorbed dose, equivalent dose and effective dose (ICRP, 2007).

Absorbed dose – SI unit: the gray (Gy)

This is a universal quantity that can be measured in material. It is a measure of the energy transferred from the radiation to the absorbing body or object, per unit mass of the absorber. This is the quantity measured by all radiation monitoring measurement instruments.

Equivalent dose – SI unit: the sievert (Sv)

Some types of ionising radiation are more hazardous than others for the same absorbed dose. For radiation risk and protection purposes therefore, a radiation weighting factor is introduced so that the relative harm of the radiation type of interest, compared with the same dose of X-rays, can be accounted for. By definition the radiation weighting factor of X-rays is 1 so, numerically, the absorbed dose and equivalent dose are the

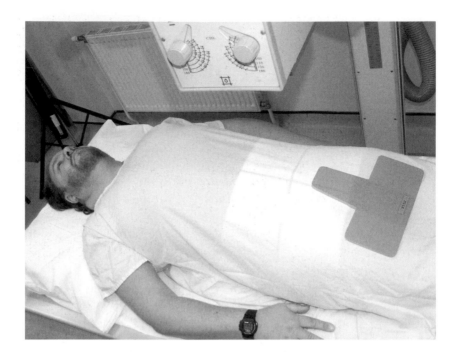

(a)

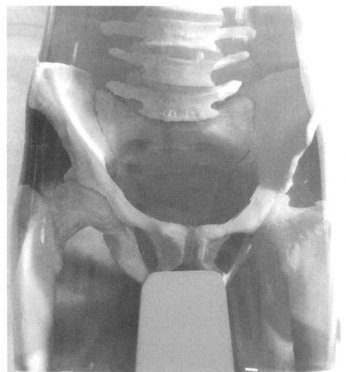

(b)

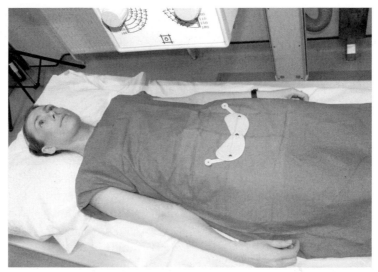

(c)

(d)

Figure 7.2 Lead rubber devices are used to shield the reproductive organs (gonads). This reduces the radiation dose to germinal tissue and thus the risk of genetic mutations that might result in hereditary radiation effects. a) Gonad protection device in position on a male patient; b) see-through (perspex and plastic) body phantom showing anatomical relationships of male gonad protection device; c) gonad protection device in position on a female patient; d) see-through (perspex and plastic) body phantom showing anatomical relationships of female gonad protection device.

same for X-rays. However, for alpha radiation the radiation weighting factor is 20, meaning that an absorbed dose of 1 Gy actually gives rise to an equivalent dose of 20 Gy. An equivalent dose is used to specify the biologically meaningful dose to a specific organ or body tissue of interest and is therefore a 'human' quantity.

Effective dose – SI unit: the sievert (Sv)

Not all organs and tissues in the human body are susceptible to the harmful effects of radiation to the same degree. In order to arrive at a dose quantity that correlates well with actual risk, account needs to be taken of the specific organs that are irradiated by introducing tissue weighting factors for all the significant organs and tissues in the body. The effective dose, incorporating both a radiation weighting factor and the tissue weighting factors in its definition, is the dose quantity that best correlates with the risk.

Both the gray and the sievert are 'large' units in the context of radiation protection. Typical doses encountered in practice are of the order of one thousandth of a gray/sievert and are thus commonly used with the prefix 'milli'; 1 millisievert (mSv) = 0.001 Sv or 10^{-3} Sv.

Measuring and estimating patient doses or 'micro' 1 microsievert (μSv) = 10^{-6} Sv

It is not possible to measure directly the radiation dose absorbed in any organ of a human body – to do so would require radiation detection devices to be embedded in and distributed throughout the whole organ, which is clearly not practical. Two quantities are commonly measured directly (NRPB, 1990) to monitor patient doses in practice: these are entrance surface dose and dose-area product.

- **Entrance surface dose (ESD)** is the absorbed dose in air (in mGy) on the surface of the patient where the centre of the X-ray beam enters the body.
- **Dose-area product (DAP)** is a compound measure of absorbed dose and area, which can be measured relatively precisely with current practical instruments, and is more meaningful than ESD for more complex examinations.

Both these measures can be converted to estimates of **effective dose** using published tables of conversion coefficients – these are based on computer simulation incorporating some assumptions about the positioning and collimation of the X-ray beam and other relevant exposure parameters (Hart *et al.*, 1994).

Records of actual DAP readings are routinely kept for all medical imaging exposures and are regularly audited to ensure they remain aligned to national dose reference levels (DRLs).

THE ADVERSE EFFECTS OF RADIATION

Any adverse effects of ionising radiation which do occur are usually apparent in those individuals who receive direct exposure. However, if the germinal tissue (namely biological tissue that is destined to form sex cells) of an individual is irradiated, it is possible that a mutation may occur in an ovum (female reproductive cell) or sperm (male reproductive cell). The effects of germinal cell mutation will be apparent in the offspring of an exposed individual if a mutated ovum or sperm cell participates in reproductive fertilisation. Radiation effects can therefore be either somatic – occurring in the exposed individual – or hereditary (genetic) – occurring in the offspring of an exposed individual. There is a further very important subdivision of radiation effects, deterministic or stochastic.

Deterministic effects

At high radiation doses, acute (early) effects known as **deterministic effects** or **tissue reactions** may occur. Above a certain threshold dose (for most effects in excess of 2 Gy) the tissue reaction will be clinically detectable, with higher radiation doses being associated with more severe effects. Below the threshold, the effect will usually be **occult** (not detectable). Examples of deterministic effects are reproductive sterility, cataract formation, skin erythema (redness) and ulceration. An adequate system of radiological protection should protect against the possibility of any of these effects in normal circumstances; however there are contemporary examples of significant tissue reactions following complex interventional fluoroscopic procedures (Shope, 1995). The time to onset of such effects can range from a few minutes to several weeks.

Stochastic effects

Stochastic effects are late effects and their probability of occurrence is related to the effective dose and is not associated with a 'threshold'. In other words, such effects are related to the radiation dose in terms of 'probability' – if the dose is doubled then the risk of such an effect occurring is also doubled. Stochastic effects include solid organ cancer and leukaemia (blood cancer). They are called late effects because, if they occur at all, they only become clinically detectable several years, or even tens of years, after exposure (ICRP, 2007).

Are low doses of ionising radiation really hazardous?

Most routine diagnostic and image-guided minimally invasive therapeutic radiation exposures are associated with low radiation doses. **Radiotherapy** doses are much higher, with the therapeutic benefit of such techniques purposefully utilising the damaging effect of radiation on abnormal (cancer) cells for clinical benefit.

The strongest evidence linking cancer development with radiation exposure comes from the medical follow-up of survivors of the Hiroshima and Nagasaki atomic bombings of 1945 (later evidence from other exposed populations is fairly consistent with this). However, direct evidence of a link between radiation exposure and cancer is only available for doses in excess of tens of milliSieverts. Estimates of risks associated with the doses typically incurred from routine diagnostic imaging procedures are inferred from these higher dose data.

In the absence of rigorous and specific evidence there is always room for alternative theories. It has been argued by some scientists that low doses of radiation are not just harmless but can be positively beneficial (Mortazavi, no date). Conversely, it has been argued by others that low doses are actually more harmful than might be suggested by simply extrapolating risk estimates from high dose data (Brenner *et al.*, 2003).

The current scientific consensus regarding stochastic (cancer) effects is that there is no threshold dose below which the probability of the effect is zero, and across the whole range of survivable radiation doses, the risk for solid cancers is directly proportional to effective dose (see Figure 7.3). For leukaemia, the relationship is not linear but curved upwards, meaning a doubling of the dose more than doubles the risk.

As a consequence, no amount of radiation exposure, however small, is considered completely safe. Having said this, it is important that the risks estimated for a given radiation exposure are kept in perspective. A radiation dose of 1 mSv, which is typical of diagnostic imaging patient exposures and the annual occupational exposures for health care staff, is associated with an estimated risk of one in 20,000 for the induction of a cancer at some time in the future. To put this into some kind of persepective it is estimated that one in three people in the UK will get cancer at some point in their life, and therefore the additional risk of getting cancer due to medical exposure to ionising radiation is very small in comparison to a person's overall risk.

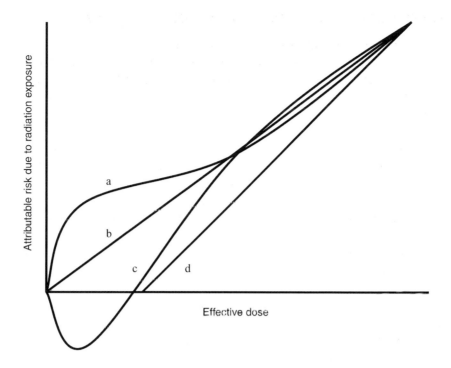

Figure 7.3 Possible dose-effect relationships for solid cancers at low doses: (a) enhanced risk at low doses; (b) linear relationship; (c) benefit at very low doses (hormesis effect); (d) threshold relationship (doses below the threshold are completely safe)

THE BENEFITS OF DIAGNOSTIC IMAGING INVESTIGATIONS

Having focused on the potential negative consequences of a medical radiation exposure, it is now time to consider the potential benefits of an imaging procedure. Although, in many cases, the benefit may seem obvious – we don't know what's wrong with a patient and we need to use radiation based imaging techniques to find out – there are, in fact, many clinical situations where a radiological investigation might be justified (see the case studies below). In some circumstances radiological examinations are justified in medico-legal investigations and for research purposes.

Case studies

When John was admitted to hospital with abdominal pain the doctors didn't know what was wrong with him and hoped that using diagnostic imaging would help them provide the answer so they could *'reach a diagnosis'*.

When Jane had abdominal pain the doctors strongly suspected it was caused by a bowel obstruction. But they were not completely certain of this as some other conditions will produce similar signs and symptoms. In Jane's case, the doctors referred her for diagnostic imaging to confirm a clinical diagnosis and *reduce/remove the degree of uncertainty* in their diagnosis.

Karen had fallen off her horse and hurt her elbow. Although the paramedics told the Accident and Emergency staff that she had a clinically obvious fracture, the specialist nurse practitioner referred Karen for radiography to *identify the extent of the injury*. Once the radiographs had revealed how complex and extensive the injury was, she transferred Karen into the care of the orthopaedic surgeons.

Rose's grandma Rita had suffered from asthma all her life. Although she seemed otherwise fit and healthy when she was admitted to hospital to have a hip replacement operation, Dr Miller the anaesthetist referred Rita for a chest X-ray to *confirm no significant abnormality*. Although he thought that nothing abnormal would show up, he had to make sure because of the potential consequences of missing something. For example, if Rita's chest had not been 'clear' it could have caused serious breathing difficulties during and immediately after her anaesthetic.

'Follow-up' diagnostic imaging investigations can provide very precise information regarding the *healing of fractures and resolution of infection, inflammation and obstruction*. A few days after Jane had been admitted onto the ward she had a repeat abdominal radiograph to *assess the size* of her bowel and to see if her obstruction was resolving. Karen also had follow-up radiographs taken six weeks after falling off her horse to assess how well her fracture was healing.

A few days after Rita's hip replacement she had radiographs taken to *confirm the position* of her hip **prosthesis**. Abdul was also waiting for radiography to confirm the position of the **internal fixation device** that had been used to pin his fractured hip. Radiography and fluoroscopy can also be used to confirm the correct positioning of **endogastric tubes**, **central venous lines** and **endovascular devices**.

Technical note

In recent decades there have been many diagnostic and therapeutic techniques developed that can be performed under fluoroscopic X-ray control or with ultrasound, CT or MRI guidance. Image-guided diagnostic and therapeutic techniques and interventional radiology procedures can sometimes save patients from having a surgical operation (see Chapter 2).

Case study

A few months after Hazel's fiftieth birthday she received a letter that told her she was now in the target population for the NHS breast screening programme. Diseases such as breast cancer represent a significant health problem in Western populations and the letter explained that although Hazel did not have any symptoms, diagnostic imaging tests such as mammography (breast radiography) could be used to 'screen for disease' and that by identifying disease at an early stage, the tests could improve **prognosis** (outcome) and reduce **morbidity** (death rate).

Hazel's screening mammogram showed some abnormal changes and, after an image-guided **biopsy** at the hospital, she was told that she did indeed have breast cancer. Dr Reynolds, the radiologist, explained that Hazel would be referred for a computed tomography (CT) examination for 'cancer staging' to provide the critical information necessary to identify if the disease had spread and to help determine the best treatment and management strategy. Dr Reynolds reassured Hazel that because the cancer had been found early there was a good chance that she could be cured.

SUMMARY: GETTING THE RISK-BENEFIT BALANCE RIGHT

Radiological investigations have many benefits – they can have a significant positive diagnostic or therapeutic impact and thus lead to improved patient management and better patient outcomes. However, they are also associated with risks – a risk of deterministic effects (tissue reactions) from high dose (mainly interventional) procedures and a risk of stochastic effects (of developing cancer at some point in the future) after any exposure to ionising radiation. The overwhelming majority of doses and risks in diagnostic imaging are small, though the risks from some high dose techniques (see Table 7.3) are certainly not negligible.

Every medical procedure involving ionising radiation needs to be individually justified and optimised. The principle of justification requires that practitioners, as defined by IR(ME)R 2000, are convinced that the potential benefit of each individual exposure outweighs its potential for harm. In order to form a rational judgement of this kind, practitioners need to have sufficient relevant knowledge, training and experience. Diagnostic radiographers typically undertake a three-year university BSc Honours degree to achieve this.

Diagnostic imaging investigation	Typical effective dose (mSv)	Equivalent number of chest X-rays	Approximate equivalent duration of natural background radiation (UK average)
General radiographic examinations			
Limbs/joints (except hip)	<0.01	<0.5	<1.5 days
Chest (single PA radiograph)	0.02	1	3 days
Skull	0.07	3	11 days
Thoracic (upper) spine	0.7	35	4 months
Lumbar (lower) spine	1.3	65	7 months
Hip	0.8	15	7 weeks
Pelvis	0.7	35	4 months
Abdomen	1.0	50	6 months
Contrast agent radiographic examinations			
Intravenous urogram (IVU)	2.5	125	14 months
Barium swallow (food pipe)	1.5	75	8 months
Barium meal (stomach)	3.0	150	16 months
Barium follow through (small intestine)	3.0	150	16 months
Barium enema (large intestine)	7.0	350	3.2 years
Computed tomography examinations			
CT – head	2.3	115	1 year
CT – chest	8	400	3.6 years
CT – abdomen or pelvis	10.0	500	4.5 years
Radionuclide imaging examinations			
Lung ventilation (Xe-133)	0.3	15	7 weeks
Lung perfusion (Tc99m)	1.0	50	6 months
Kidney (Tc99m)	1.0	50	6 months
Thyroid (Tc99m)	1.0	50	6 months
Bone (Tc99m)	4	200	1.8 years
Dynamic cardiac (Tc99m)	6.0	300	2.7 years
PET head (F18)	5.0	250	2.3 years

Table 7.3 Effective doses for a range of common diagnostic imaging investigations (RCR, 2007)

Having determined that a procedure involving the use of ionising radiation is justified, practitioners and operators must then make every effort to perform the procedure in a dose efficient manner. This means keeping the radiation dose at the lowest practicable level that is consistent with the diagnostic/therapeutic requirements of the procedure. Radiographers who undertake more complex or specialist imaging procedures usually have to undergo further postgraduate training before they can perform these examinations safely.

FURTHER READING

Allisy-Roberts, P.J. and Williams, J. (2008) *Farr's Physics for Medical Imaging* (2nd Ed). Philadelphia: Saunders, Elsevier
Chapter 2: Radiation Hazards and Protection covers radiation protection issues.

Martin, J. and Sutton, D.G. (2006) *Practical Radiation Protection in Health Care*. Oxford: Oxford University Press
Explains all aspects of radiation in detail for those who want to know more about dose measurement and safety issues.

Statkiewicz, M.A., Visconti, P.J. and Ritenour, E.R. (2006) *Radiation Protection in Medical Radiography* (5th Ed). London: Mosby
A well-written, easy to understand reference text with excellent tables, graphs and illustrations.

Chapter 8

Requesting and Reporting Imaging Investigations

Anne-Marie Dixon and Gary Culpan

INTRODUCTION

Most people will have at least one 'medical imaging' investigation at some time in their lives. Earlier chapters have explained how medical imaging can be used to diagnose disease in patients with symptoms, to screen people without symptoms for early (hidden) disease and to guide needles into the body to obtain samples or give treatment. Patients should be referred to medical imaging health care professionals for investigations to confirm or refute a clinical diagnosis based on a patient's physical signs and symptoms and/or their biochemical (blood and urine) test results. After the examination, medical imaging health care professionals will return patients to the referrer, with a **report** of the medical imaging investigation, for further management and care.

REQUESTING MEDICAL IMAGING INVESTIGATIONS

Patients are typically **referred** for medical imaging investigations when an imaging **request** is raised and forwarded to the imaging department. Traditionally, a doctor would write out a request card and send it to the imaging department. These days requests and examination appointments are more commonly administered electronically.

The imaging request has legal status and has several functions. Initially the imaging request is a formal means of transferring medical care, albeit temporarily, from one clinician (namely, the patient's general practitioner or hospital consultant) to another, for example the radiologist (GMC, 1998). The imaging request also serves as a legal prescription to administer radiation, and any associated pharmaceuticals, including a radionuclide or radiographic contrast agent, to an individual. Last, but not least, the imaging request communicates important clinical information to the radiologist, which will help ensure each patient gets the most appropriate medical imaging investigation and that the referrer gets a useful report of that examination.

Before starting a medical imaging examination, the information in the referral is checked with the patient to make sure it is accurate and complete. Where discrepancies exist, an examination may be delayed while the referrer is contacted for clarification.

The Royal College of Radiologists provides guidance on which investigations are most appropriate for a range of clinical signs and suspected pathologies, to assist those with responsibility for patient management who are considering referring patients for medical imaging investigations. *Making the Best Use of Clinical Radiology Services* (RCR, 2007) is the latest version of this guidance. Unless local protocols exist to the contrary, radiographers and radiologists may decline to perform investigations that do not comply with this guidance.

The NHS Plan (2000) recognises that patient care is improved when doctors and other health care professionals work in **multidisciplinary teams** where health care tasks are performed by those with the appropriate skills and knowledge irrespective of their individual professional status. Implementation of the NHS Plan over the last few years has involved creative skills-mix initiatives that have allowed nurses and allied health professionals (such as radiographers) to advance their practice and extend their roles to undertake some tasks that were traditionally only performed by doctors. As such, doctors can now formally **delegate** responsibility for referring patients for medical imaging investigations to non-medically qualified personnel such as nurses and physiotherapists (RCN, 2007), and radiologists can delegate medical imaging examination reporting to radiographers and nurses (RCR/SoR, 2007).

Case study

Rukhsana, the clinical nurse specialist in Accident and Emergency (A&E), and Errol, a senior radiographer, were preparing a case to go to the hospital's 'Advanced Practice Steering Group', so that they could set up a Minor Injuries Unit where Rukhsana would be able to request radiographic examinations and Errol would be able to report them. In their introduction, they tried to convince the Group that this would improve patient care – their main reason being that this 'New Way of Working' would reduce the time that patients spent in A&E because they would only wait to see the doctor once and, when they did, they would already have had their X-ray examination and would have obtained the results.

As part of their case, Rukhsana and Errol had developed local protocols, guidelines and a written **Scheme of Work** that specified which patients and types of injury were covered by the new system, and which members of staff would be involved. They provided evidence that they had both undergone appropriate training and had been assessed as competent to undertake the delegated roles, and they outlined the training and assessment criteria for any colleagues who also might like to extend their role in future. Mr Matthews, the A&E consultant, and Dr Stevens, the radiologist, were both named in the proposal as the medical practitioners who retained overall responsibility for the patients, and both Rukhsana's and Errol's line managers were named as supporters of the initiative.

After reading the proposal and listening to a short supporting presentation, the Advanced Practice Steering Group were satisfied that the proposal was achievable; they were convinced it would improve services for patients and also believed it would improve staff morale and help retain experienced senior staff like Rukhsana and Errol. The Group made a recommendation that the proposal be accepted and, a few weeks later, Rukhsana and Errol received formal written agreement from their employing hospital Trust, along with revised job descriptions that incorporated their new roles and responsibilities.

Technical note

Health care workers are professionally accountable, and their employers are legally liable (against civil suits for negligence or criminal prosecutions for intent to harm), for core competence activities, namely those activities for which they were originally trained and assessed. Nurses and allied health care professionals may undertake role extension activities, and thus perform tasks that are traditionally the responsibility of others, providing they do so under formally agreed Schemes of Work that are approved by their employing authority. As long as individual health care workers practise within the Scheme of Work, the employing Trust will provide legal indemnity. Health care practitioners remain individually accountable to their professional and registration bodies (for example, the Society of Radiographers and the Health Professions Council or Nursing and Midwifery Council), and must adhere to the professional and statutory Codes of Conduct.

REPORTING MEDICAL IMAGING INVESTIGATIONS

A request for a medical imaging investigation is not so much a request for images, but more a request for an interpretation of those same images.

Occasionally specialists within a hospital do get to see the actual images and, when viewing them either on a TV monitor or on a traditional viewing box, it is important that the viewing conditions are optimised as they would be for formal image reporting within the medical imaging department. As most medical images, and the pathologies contained therein, are displayed in grey-scale, it is important to reduce the ambient lighting (using dimmer switches) and to mask any areas of extraneous light around the image, either electronically on the monitor (shuttering) or physically on a viewing box, so that the human eye can detect the subtle differences in image contrast.

Particularly in an Accident and Emergency department, when images that have not been formally reported are viewed by referring clinicians, radiographers may participate in a **'red dot' system**. In such a system, images are annotated with a red dot or another identifying mark, to indicate when the radiographer suspects that an abnormality is shown on the image.

In most cases, however, the end-product of a medical imaging investigation is a formal examination report produced in the medical imaging department. Once added to the patient's official record, this is the permanent legal record of the imaging examination (RCR, 1999). In addition to being the official record of the examination, the report has an immediate and important role in communicating information about the patient's health status, which will have been discovered during the medical imaging procedure, to those responsible for that patient's care. Thus the medical imaging report will typically contain a 'description' of the anatomical or functional appearances demonstrated during the imaging procedure, as well as an 'interpretation' of what these appearances mean for the patient in terms of health or illness. Sometimes, the imaging report will contain 'recommendations' for further tests and investigations, or may perhaps suggest a particular course of treatment.

From the above, it is clear that those who compile medical imaging investigation reports need to have a wide range of clinical and technical medical imaging knowledge. Traditionally, medical image reporting has been performed by radiologists and their professional body (the Royal College of Radiologists) includes guidance on report content and communication in their 'Good Practice' guidelines (RCR, 1999). In recent years however, demand for medical imaging tests has increased to such a level that there are not enough radiologists to report imaging investigations in a timely and clinically efficient manner, and so radiographers (and, in some hospitals, nurses) have also been trained to undertake this role. As with image requesting, radiographer or nurse reporting is considered a **role extension** activity; it must be undertaken under a formal system of **delegation** (RCR/ SoR, 2007) and performed to the same standard as radiologist reporting.

Results of imaging investigations may be communicated verbally, particularly when urgent treatment is indicated, but all medical imaging investigations should have some form of permanent report. Most often, a written report is created and communicated to the person requesting the investigation. In simplest terms this may be a handwritten entry in a patient's case notes, but more usually it is a separate document. Traditionally, a paper copy of an imaging investigation report would be posted to the referrer to be inserted into the patient's notes. Increasingly health care institutions are keeping patient records electronically and thus soft copy reports are created, circulated, stored and linked entirely within computerised systems such as *PACS*. Access to such systems, and indeed to paper versions of patient records, is governed by the Data Protection Act (HMSO, 1999) and restricted to authorised persons; electronic records are usually kept on secure password protected systems or can only be accessed using individually issued SMART cards.

In some cases, imaging reports are placed in hand-held notes that the patient carries around with them. This is common practice in antenatal care where a pregnant woman has a file or booklet in which her obstetrician, midwife and other health carers, such as the sonographer, can record the results of physical examinations, blood tests and ultrasound scans. This practice is also becoming more common as **one-stop clinics** are introduced where a patient gets a series of tests at one attendance and carries the results around until they finally hand them to the doctor who will discuss all of these with the patient and her family or other accompanying supporters.

Ultimately, it is the responsibility of the referring clinician to convey any information about the medical imaging investigation results to the patient. Although it is frustrating for patients when they are denied information about the results at the time of the examination, the radiographers and radiologists performing those examinations will often have only a limited clinical knowledge of the patient and are not in a position to fully discuss the implications of the results; in almost all cases they will also not have responsibility for clinical management.

Report content

One of the first things a medical imaging report must contain is enough information to identify it as belonging to one specific individual patient and to relate it to one specific episode of care. Typically the report will contain the patient's name, at least one other piece of unique identifying information such as their hospital or NHS number, and the dates that the imaging investigation was performed and the report compiled (if different). All this information should be checked first by anyone reading the report, as the report is useless, if not even dangerous, if it is interpreted as relating to an incorrect patient or a different examination occurrence.

Medical imaging reports should also contain the name of the person who has referred the patient for the investigation – this information is useful for clerical staff so that they know who to send the report to (and who to charge for the investigation if it is performed under private health care arrangements), but it is also useful to other people reading the report as it usually indicates who has overall **clinical responsibility** for the patient (GMC, 2006). In addition, whoever is compiling the report needs to know who is likely to read it, in order that the language and terminology they use can be pitched at a level that makes the information understandable and informative (RCR, 1999). If the request comes from a patient's General Practitioner, the report may include a recommendation for hospital referral; clearly this would not be necessary if the request had come from a hospital consultant in the first place and a recommendation for further management may be inappropriate in such cases.

Although there are general recommendations about the technical and clinical information that should be contained in an imaging investigation report, local protocols and/or standardised reports, or proformas, should be developed between those requesting and reporting examinations to cover routinely required information. Particular care needs to be taken when compiling reports to go in patients' hand-held notes as the patient concerned will be able to read these. Local protocols may therefore contain 'coded phrases' that can be used to avoid alarming the patient while still conveying important diagnostic information between health care workers.

Case study

Albert had recently been invited to attend an aortic aneurysm screening programme. The referral letter from his GP had confirmed Albert was over 65 years of age and, as a male, he met the criteria to join the screening programme. As such, Albert was invited for serial ultrasound scans, every 6–12 months, to measure the diameter of his aorta (the main artery carrying blood to the abdomen and legs).

After the first screening examination Sally, the radiographer, ticked the report proforma to indicate that Albert's aorta was widened (25–50 mm diameter). Mr Siddique, the vascular surgeon, read the report and then told Albert that if it got wider than 50 mm, or extended to affect the blood flow to his kidneys or legs, he would recommend an operation or image-guided interventional procedure to minimise the risk of his aorta leaking or bursting.

Technical note

Abdominal aortic aneurysm (AAA) is particularly prevalent in older men and has a significant risk of death. Sometimes asymptomatic AAAs are discovered incidentally when performing imaging investigations for unrelated signs and symptoms. Structured screening programmes, such as the one Albert was invited to, are currently being evaluated in the elderly male population to see if they are cost-effective. A minimally invasive procedure done in the imaging department, aortic stenting (see Chapter 2), can strengthen the aorta and stop it from leaking or bursting. A ruptured aortic aneurysm is often a clinical emergency requiring a major operation – and many patients do not survive.

As a communication from one health care individual to another, the imaging examination report's content and interpretation will depend on these two people having a mutual understanding of the other's perspective. Those requesting imaging investigations need to give enough background and clinical information in referrals in order that those writing reports can produce an accurate, explicit and unambiguous interpretation (RCR, 1999).

Initially, the body of the report should contain a brief summary of the clinical information given on the request card by the referrer – essentially this tells the reader what conditions the clinician is expecting the imaging investigation to confirm or refute.

The report should then contain a statement about what investigation has actually been performed and any specialist techniques, such as **contrast agent** administration or additional projections/sequences, which have been employed. If the normal imaging examination protocol has not been followed, or any difficulties have been encountered during the examination, these limitations should also be mentioned in the report (RCR, 1999).

The clinical part of the report should describe the anatomical structures/physiological processes examined and the investigation findings: this might include a description of their appearances, an interpretation of whether these are considered normal or pathological, and some comment comparing the current investigation results to any obtained previously. The report should only contain specialist technical language or terminology that the reader is likely to understand. Sometimes a reference will be made to charts, graphs or tables to check if structures are of a normal size or whether physiological measurements are within normal limits. Charts and graphs are particularly used in ultrasound scanning to check the size and growth of unborn babies and it is important that both the reporters and the referrers know which charts are being used and that they are appropriate for the local population.

The body of the report should conclude with a diagnosis, or short list of likely alternative or **differential diagnoses**. This section of the report should be worded in a way that conveys to the reader the level of certainty the reporter has in their conclusion and, where indicated, further tests and investigations may be recommended to confirm or clarify the imaging findings (RCR, 1999).

Finally, the report should contain the name and professional status of the health care worker who has compiled the report, and the date on which this was done. When a particular imaging health care professional has had significant involvement in performing a more complex examination, their name and status should also be included in the report.

Although the medical imaging report is often considered the definitive 'result' of an investigation, it must be remembered that it is essentially a professional opinion and, as such, there will inevitably be an element of variability between the individuals producing such reports: in most cases this may essentially lie only in the report's style, with reporting accuracy being assured if it is performed by an appropriately trained individual.

Case study

Angela, the sonographer, was careful to read Arthur's carotid ultra-sound referral and his hospital notes before doing his examination. Angela started her examination report with a brief summary of Arthur's symptoms (dizzy spells) and a statement that she was aiming to confirm Mr Siddique's impression that Arthur had a carotid stenosis. Angela then stated that she had performed a standard 'carotid ultrasound' examination with no complications or limitations. The report then went on to list the blood flow velocities in the carotid vessels and concluded with Angela's diagnosis that there was no signif-icant stenosis. Finally, Angela made a recommendation that Arthur have a computed tomography (CT) scan to see if the dizzy spells were caused by an abnormality in his brain.

Technical note

Although many imaging investigations are performed according to stan-dardised protocols, armed with the details of each patient's specific situation, reporters can pay special attention to making sure the exam-ination report is as informative as possible and is tailored specifically to each individual patient.

Learning activity

Every imaging report is different – each is customised to an individual examination of a specific person on one particular occasion – and each imaging department has its own style and format for producing examination reports – these are agreed between referring and reporting clinical staff. Next time you get the opportunity on a clinical placement ask to have a look at some imaging investigation reports and see if you can identify all the relevant information described in this chapter.

SUMMARY

Medical imaging investigations are performed on patients suspected to have, or to be at risk of, a clinical abnormality and are only indicated when the result is reasonably expected to have an influence on patient management. Traditionally, medical imaging investigations were performed when one doctor referred a patient temporarily to the specialist care of another. Over the last few years patient care has been improved by encouraging the delegation of referral duties to suitably trained registered nurses and allied health professionals.

The result of a medical imaging investigation is invariably contained in a formal report that forms part of a patient's official legal record. Medical imaging examination reporting, traditionally the task of a radiologist, is also now often delegated to suitably trained and registered non-medical health care professionals to facilitate the timely and clinically efficient communication of the results.

The appropriate delegation of referral and reporting responsibilities is undertaken within formal Schemes of Work, where employing hospital Trusts will authorise individual practitioners to extend their roles and advance their practice. Medical imaging investigation referrals and reports are legal documents and vital tools for communicating pertinent information between health care professionals caring for patients. As such they must be completed with due care and attention.

FURTHER READING

Dimond, B. (2002) *Legal Aspects of Radiography and Radiology.* Oxford: Blackwell

Chapter 9

Looking After Those Who Need Imaging Examinations
Terry Lodge and Anne-Marie Dixon

INTRODUCTION

A person may have a diagnostic medical imaging examination either as an out-patient or as a ward or in-patient. They may be referred by their General Practitioner (GP), they may present themselves at hospital following an accident, for example, or they may be invited to participate in a screening programme or research investigation. While in the imaging department, that person will be cared for by a **multidisciplinary team** of health professionals, all of whom will have had special training in the technical aspects of performing diagnostic imaging examinations and image-guided procedures. The **radiographers, radiologists**, nurses and other support staff in the imaging department will have also had professional training in how to look after, support and care for people during these examinations and procedures. Their responsibilities will include effective communication, ensuring safety, promoting well-being, and preserving dignity and autonomy. They will always try to adopt a person- or family-centred approach.

A person undergoing imaging investigations may be either permanently or temporarily dependent on the health care professionals looking after them. In this vulnerable state they will have a right to expect that their health care professionals will act as advocates and guardians. Care responsibilities will start before the imaging examination itself, will continue during the procedure, and will even extend until after the results have been dispatched.

CARE RESPONSIBILITIES BEFORE THE EXAMINATION

Person/family-centred care

Radiographers and other imaging department staff will usually have limited contact with people having imaging investigations, and any accompanying supporters such as family or friends, immediately before a procedure. During this time the radiographer will have to formally meet and identify the person undergoing the investigation, and then commence a dialogue and establish a rapport that will gain the person's confidence and help them understand the procedure and their role in its success.

When first meeting the person who is having the examination, the radiographer will have to assess their physical and mental capacity in order that they can adapt their care and radiographic technique to meet that person's individual needs. With the best will and professionalism in the world, during this limited contact time before an examination radiographers simply do not have sufficient opportunity to gain a full understanding of everyone's personal issues, fears and expectations. When friends and relatives, or other health care professionals such as nurses, accompany people to the imaging department they will have far more knowledge about that person and their circumstances than the radiographer can ever be aware of. Therefore, as well as communicating with the person having the imaging investigation, a radiographer will also have to consider the contribution that those accompanying that person can make.

Pre-test anxiety

When someone is initially referred for an imaging examination they may have little accurate knowledge of what such a procedure will entail. Each individual may have their own ideas about what to expect, but if that person has no prior personal experience then any expectation is likely to be based on what they might have read, seen on television or been told by other people – and usually such representations are far from the truth and often have a negative bias. Fear of the unknown is a recognised source of anxiety, but no matter how long or how many times someone may have been in an imaging department and however comfortable and socialised they might feel with hospital routines, each visit will present a new source of anxiety.

If someone coming for an imaging investigation is unduly nervous about the actual procedure it might make them less likely to be able to comply with even the simplest instructions given to them by the imaging department staff. Radiographers can recognise that some people are confused by their unfamiliar surroundings, that they find the equipment and even the health care staff intimidating, and that they might be fearful to some extent about the consequences of the test results or worried about the possibility of diagnosis of a serious condition. Fear of a 'negative' examination (when nothing abnormal is found) is also recognised as distressing as it means the cause of symptoms has not been established. People who are in pain or otherwise disoriented may also be anxious that they will not be able to tolerate the procedure or comply with the required instructions.

A patient who has been well informed about what to expect, particularly if this has been done before the actual visit, will be less likely to be worried about the procedure and will therefore be more likely to be receptive to instructions and prepared to do their best to comply with them. The administrative and professional staff in an imaging department will try to greet people coming to them for investigations with a friendly face and will be prepared to spend some time giving explanations and reassurance. However, it is much better if fear can be allayed and anxiety minimised in advance, through the transmission of suitable information and explanations by those other health care staff who have been involved in referring for imaging and supporting people thorough their health care journey.

Information leaflets

Imaging departments usually have a ready supply of general and examination-specific leaflets that can give a broad overview of the purpose of various investigations, as well as the details of any specific preparation requirements before attending, and that will include practical information about what will happen, when and where (see Figure 9.1).

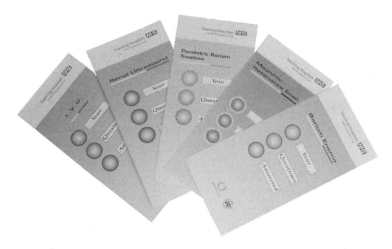

Figure 9.1 A selection of typical information leaflets that might be sent out with imaging examination appointment letters

Quite commonly, people will be asked to restrict their diet before attending for imaging investigations or they will be told that they may need to take medicines or drink water before they attend (details of those examinations that require periods of starvation, laxative administration or bladder filling, have been given in earlier chapters). It is important that people understand why these requirements are essential to the procedure and will be fundamental to a successful examination that produces a diagnostically accurate result. A supply of information leaflets may be held and given out by those health carers responsible for making the imaging investigation referrals, but they are also commonly sent out or incorporated with appointment letters. Such leaflets will include a contact telephone number so that additional information or clarification can be obtained if necessary.

Just before the actual examination, the radiographer will give a detailed verbal explanation of the procedure to convey an understanding of what action and behaviours are required for an optimal and successful examination: this helps to prevent the need for repeat exposures and thus an unnecessary radiation dose.

Getting to the imaging department

Information leaflets and appointment letters will contain information about, and often a map of, the geographic location of the institution where the imaging procedure will take place. It is not unusual for this to be in a separate building or even another hospital to the one originally attended. In addition, careful consideration will need to be taken regarding the mode of transport that will be used.

Case study

Margaret was quite indignant when Bob the porter came up to the ward to take her down to the imaging department for a chest X-ray. She said she had been told that maintaining her independence for as long as possible would help to keep her fit and well in the future. Margaret claimed she was perfectly able to walk and refused to sit in the wheelchair. Sister Wells came over to see what the fuss was about and calmly explained that the hospital had a policy that required everyone to be transferred between wards and other departments using hospital transport devices such as wheelchairs and hospital trolleys. Bob then explained that it was his job to ensure Margaret got to and from the imaging department safely and, with Sister Wells' agreement, if she felt OK on the way back she could walk some of the way.

Professional note

Where a patient can stand or sit safely for a period of time a wheelchair is the most appropriate form of transport. Patients who cannot stand safely, and those who cannot be moved around without causing them significant pain, should attend the department on a trolley.

Hospital trolleys are used for people who have suffered severe accidental trauma and those who have had major surgery recently. Some trolleys have been specially designed for use in Accident and Emergency departments so the image detector can be positioned in a tray incorporated below the trolley mattress (see Figure 9.2).

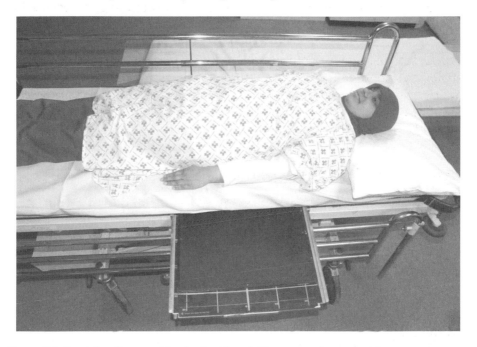

Figure 9.2 Special trolleys used in the Accident & Emergency department incorporate a tray under the mattress so the X-ray detector plate can be positioned without having to move a severely injured patient onto an X-ray examination table

On rare occasions it may be necessary for immobile patients to be transported to (and from) the imaging department in their hospital bed. In such circumstances this will then only require the patient to be moved twice (from their bed to the imaging couch and back again) or it may be possible for the patient to have their examination without being moved from their bed.

It is possible to undertake radiographic examinations of severely ill or infectious patients on a hospital ward (see Figure 9.3a and b). Mobile or bedside radiography is important in **intensive care** and **coronary care** units, where patients may be unconscious on a breathing machine (ventilator) or may need to have their heart function continuously monitored, and in **isolation** units where patients are having **barrier nursing**. However, the quality of images and the range of examinations that can be undertaken at the bedside are very limited; in addition, such examinations may

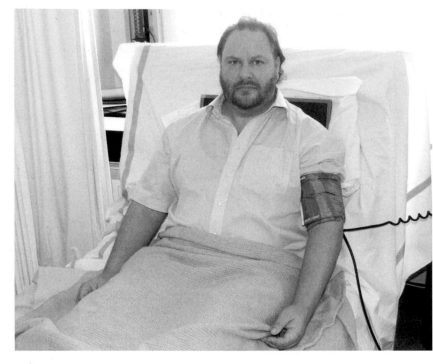

(a)

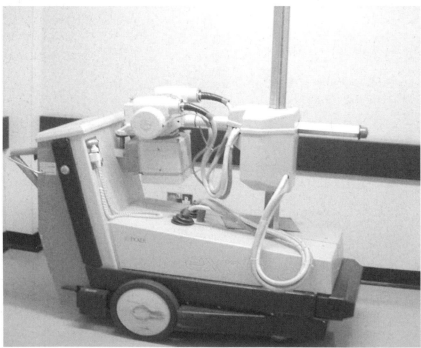

(b)

Figure 9.3 (a) Patients who are attached to monitoring equipment can be X-rayed on the ward (b) using small mobile machines if absolutely necessary

expose the ward staff and other patients to unnecessary radiation. Requests for mobile radiography are not routine and each will need to be discussed individually with the imaging department's staff.

People attending for imaging investigations from home will generally walk, drive or get to hospital as a passenger by car, bus, train or taxi. Elderly and disabled people may be entitled to ambulance transport. As explained in earlier chapters, some imaging investigations will require injections and/or the administration of contrast agents and, where appropriate, people will be warned in advance if this means that they should not drive home following the procedure.

Examination gowns

Case study

Before Paul had abdominal radiography he was asked to change out of his normal outer clothing and wear a hospital examination gown. (See Figure 9.4). Evelyn, the health care assistant, explained that this plain cotton garment did not have any buttons, zips or pockets (to contain things) that might show up on the images. Once Paul had removed his own clothes and put the gown on he felt a bit vulnerable and exposed – he was glad he had been told to bring his own dressing gown to wear on top. Paul was relieved when Evelyn showed him to a small private waiting area.

Professional note

Hospital examination gowns are used for many imaging investigations so the images are free from artefacts. Being able to bring their own dressing gown helps to preserve a person's self-identity; imaging department staff will take great care to ensure that people who are not in their normal clothes can wait in areas that will preserve their dignity and privacy.

Someone who has already been admitted to a hospital ward (an in-patient) may already be in a hospital gown. However, radiographers recognise that they may be ill-at-ease in their new 'patient uniform', may be struggling to come to terms with their illness and may be somewhat disorientated by the many different staff, hospital departments and tests that they are encountering.

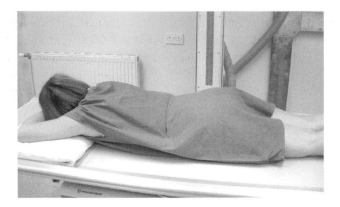

(a)

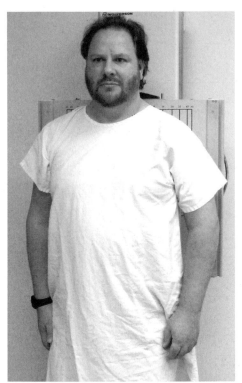

(b)

Figure 9.4 (a) and (b) Patients will usually be asked to change into plain cotton hospital examination gowns to prevent metallic objects appearing on their images

Questions, questions and more questions!

One of the things that tends to annoy people visiting hospitals is the number of questions they are asked and the number of times the same questions are asked repeatedly. However, poor systems or a failure to adhere to the appropriate systems of checking patient and examination details can lead to professional mistakes, some of which will have potentially devastating consequences. In the simplest terms, irradiating the 'wrong' patient is considered legally to be 'assault'; all radiation exposures are associated with some risk of adverse effects (see Chapter 7) and performing an interventional procedure on, or administering contrast agents to, the wrong patient may, in a worst case scenario, cause death. Most of the questioning is therefore essential to the processes of identification, justification and optimisation and is also required under the Ionising Radiation (Medical Exposures) Regulations 2000 (see Chapter 7).

Identification protocols

At the outset of any imaging procedure the radiographer must obtain a positive identification. This involves asking an individual for information that will identify them as the person to be examined. The details that are usually requested will be a person's name, date of birth and address, and these will then be checked against the information in the imaging referral (see Figure 9.5). Wherever possible this information must come from the individual themselves – when someone cannot speak for themselves the imaging department staff will check their identification band and/or verify their patient identification with their accompanying supporters or ward staff. If a person cannot be positively identified, or any discrepancies exist in the referral documentation, the imaging examination will not be performed.

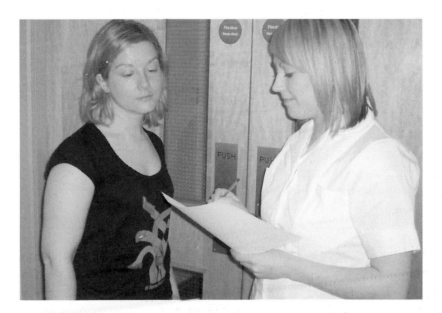

Figure 9.5 The radiographer will carefully check a person's name, address and date of birth before taking them for an imaging investigation

The '28 day' and '10 day' rules

To prevent the unnecessary irradiation of an unborn baby, when imaging procedures involve irradiation of the reproductive organs of females of child bearing age (usually defined as between the ages of 12 and 55 years) they will be asked if there is any possibility that they could be pregnant. Female members of staff who are required to assist during ionising radiation examinations will also be asked this question.

Case study

Andrea was a bit surprised when Sally asked her if there was any possibility that she could be pregnant, once she had closed the door after bringing her into the X-ray room, but she was glad she had been asked the question somewhere confidential and private. When Andrea said that she didn't think she was pregnant, Sally asked her if she could remember the first date of her last menstrual period. Andrea remembered that she had had a period the week before and when Sally heard this she explained that it would be OK to go ahead with the examination.

Professional note

A woman will normally be considered 'not pregnant' and the imaging investigation can go ahead if she is within 28 days from starting her last menstrual period – the '28 day rule'. For some high dose and therefore higher risk examinations a woman is considered potentially pregnant once she has passed the ovulation phase of her menstrual cycle: high dose examinations will usually only be performed in the first 10 days of a woman's menstrual cycle – the '10 day rule'.

Imaging examinations of pregnant women are only carried out after a careful consideration of the risks and benefits to both mother and baby. In addition, general health care staff members who are pregnant are usually excluded from the room while imaging investigations involving ionising radiation are performed.

Allergies and other contraindications

Prior to the administration of **contrast agents** people will be asked if they suffer from any allergies. Positive responses will alert the imaging department staff to an increased risk of allergic reaction to an intravenously administered iodine-based contrast agent. Because of adverse affects on renal function, Metformin® therapy (usually for diabetes) is temporarily withdrawn when iodine-based contrast agents are to be administered. (Allergies and contraindications are discussed in detail in Chapter 2.)

Previous imaging investigations

People are asked if they have had previous imaging tests for several reasons. Firstly, it helps a radiographer assess how much knowledge a person might have about what is going to happen and they can tailor their explanation accordingly. The information is also an important aspect of the justification process to ensure that the diagnostic information has not already been obtained, either from the same test performed earlier or through an alternative test. Imaging department staff will also need to look at images and reports from previous examinations to see if there are any features (anatomical or **pathological**) that might require them to modify the examination. In addition, when the examination report is being compiled current images will be compared with previous ones in order that comments can be made about any deterioration or improvement. Although checks for previous examinations are routinely made by clerical staff when referrals are received, when examinations have been performed at other hospitals or people have changed their name or address, records might not be matched up. The concept of the **electronic patient record** – a centrally stored national database of patient information – is part of the government's National Programme for Information Technology (Health Committee, 2007). The aim of the Programme is to facilitate the sharing of data between institutions and thus speed up communication and reduce the likelihood of clinical errors, features that should consequently improve service efficiency and patient safety.

Informed consent

As in all other areas of health care, gaining informed consent is essential before starting any imaging procedure. The principle of informed consent respects the right of an individual to determine what happens to their own body. Failure to obtain valid consent may render a health care professional liable to legal or disciplinary action (DoH, 2001).

Provision of adequate information is an essential prerequisite for giving informed consent. Before a person can consent to undergo an imaging procedure they need to have a description of what to expect, an explanation of how the examination will benefit them, some idea of why this particular examination is better than any alternative one, and an overview of any significant risks or side effects.

In many situations consent for an imaging procedure is obtained verbally as an agreement to proceed once the examination has been explained, and it is not formally recorded. However, for some complex and/or invasive procedures and those associated with significant risk and/or side effects, a written consent form will be completed (GMC, 1998) (see Figure 9.6). Formal written consent is also obtained for examinations (or use of images and/or results) that are not primarily associated with clinical care, such as when used for teaching or research purposes (GMC, 1998). Although not a legal requirement, it is considered good practice to make people aware when student practitioners will be observing, assisting or conducting imaging examinations (DoH, 2001).

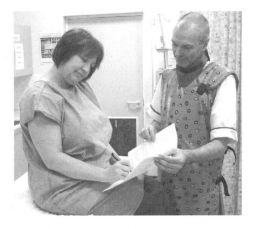

Figure 9.6 For some complex examinations or for invasive procedures patients will be asked to sign a consent form

CARE RESPONSIBILITIES DURING IMAGING EXAMINATIONS

Many imaging examinations are of short duration and afford only a very short period of contact time between radiographers and the people having the investigations. For most of this time, the radiographer will be concentrating on the technical aspects of the examination that have been discussed in earlier chapters of this book. Nevertheless, radiographers are not just 'technicians' – they are professional health care staff and are also aware of their extended responsibilities to look after and care for the people who come to them, albeit temporarily, for investigation or treatment. Radiographers may seek the assistance of a person's accompanying supporters, such as their family, friends, carers and other hospital staff, when performing imaging investigations and procedures.

Accompanying supporters

For many examinations it is usual for accompanying supporters to be asked to stay outside the imaging room during the actual examination. This is to protect people from the hazardous effects of radiation, but it also affords the person having the examination a degree of privacy, particularly if personal questions (about pregnancy or the signs and symptoms of their illness) are being asked. When people are waiting before, during and after the investigation, their supporters and other health care staff will usually be allowed to wait with them.

Case study

Amjid had brought his four-year-old son Ali for an X-ray of his arm after he had fallen off his bike. Sally, the radiographer, explained that she would need Amjid to stay with Ali while he had his X-ray to help reassure him and keep him still. Ali thought his dad looked funny in the lead rubber apron that Sally had given him to wear but he stopped crying when he realised he wouldn't be left on his own. Ali tried really hard to keep still for his dad although his arm was hurting quite a bit. He kept very still and quiet and listened for the 'beeping' noise that Sally said he would hear when she was taking his picture.

Professional note

When small children, vulnerable adults, or those with learning difficulties are being imaged, a parent or other relative or carer will usually be allowed to remain in the examination room: the presence and encouragement of a familiar face can be important to the success of the examination. Sometimes these people are asked to stand with the radiographer by the control panel, safely behind a protective lead-glass or lead-lined screen (see Figure 9.7). If they need to remain close and in view, they will be asked to wear lead rubber protective clothing similar to that sometimes worn by imaging staff (see Figure 9.8).

Chaperones

For some imaging examinations, particularly those of an intimate nature such as barium enema (see Chapter 2) or transvaginal ultrasound (see Chapter 5), the presence of a chaperone should be offered (RCR, 1998). This is particularly important for female patients if the radiographer or radiologist is male (see Figure 9.9) but chaperone use irrespective of the health carer's gender is considered good general practice (SoR, 2007) as it promotes a sense of well-being and is a gesture of respect. Chaperones should be members of the clinical team who know enough about the

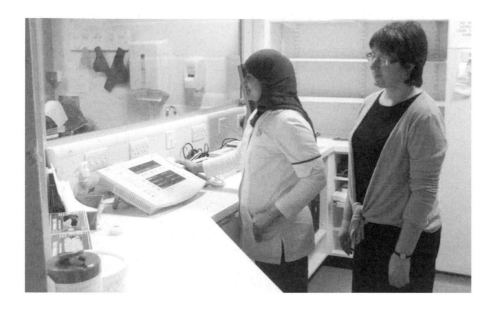

Figure 9.7 When a patient's relative has to stay in the X-ray room to ensure the co-operation of the patient, the relative will be asked to stand behind the lead glass control panel screen with the radiographer while the actual exposure is made so that they do not receive an unnecessary radiation dose

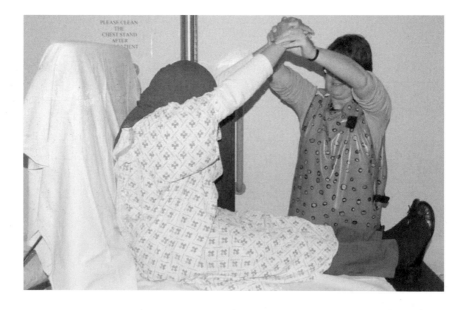

Figure 9.8 Where patients are unable to keep still or cannot support themselves in the correct position, relatives will sometimes be asked to wear a lead rubber apron and assist. While the associated radiation dose is minimal, this does prevent health care staff repeatedly performing the task and accumulating an unacceptable radiation dose

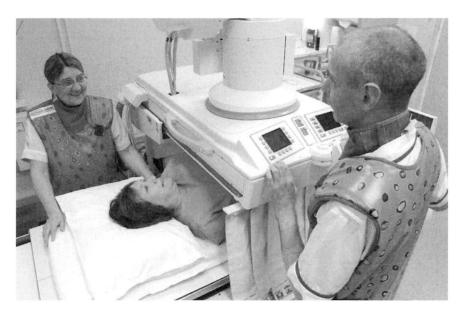

Figure 9.9 Chaperones are routinely used for 'intimate' examinations – in particular a female patient will be offered a female chaperone when being examined by a male radiographer or radiologist

examinations to judge whether or not they are being performed appropriately.

Cross infection

It is important that the imaging department is told of any contagious medical conditions or infections such as MRSA (methicillin resistant Staphylococcus aureus) that may be transferred to other people. While all members of staff will have been trained in effective hand washing and will clean imaging equipment and accessories between procedures, it may be necessary to carry out additional disinfection and, in some cases, sterilisation processes, after people with contagious conditions have been imaged. Additional infection control measures will also be undertaken prior to imaging people who are **immunocompromised** (at increased risk of infection) if the department is made aware of this in advance.

Repeat imaging

Probably the most stressful thing that can happen to people who have had their imaging investigation and are waiting to be told they can leave, is being asked to come back into the room for 'one more picture'. The most common reason for additional imaging is that the original examination did not demonstrate the required anatomy and further views/

projections are required in a different position or using different exposure factors. Sometimes image quality does not reach the standard required for optimal diagnostic accuracy for a variety of technical (and occasionally human) reasons, and the same imaging is then repeated to get a satisfactory level of diagnostic quality. While radiographers are usually not at liberty to divulge imaging test results directly (see Chapter 8), they will try to attempt to reassure and empathise with people, and are being honest when they try to dispel feelings that repeat imaging must mean that 'something bad' has been seen.

CARE RESPONSIBILITIES AFTER IMAGING EXAMINATIONS

Aftercare

Once people have been informed that their imaging examination is finished, most will be told that they can simply get changed into their normal clothes and return home or to the ward, and that they will experience no side effects. However, some imaging procedures do require specialist aftercare and these have been described in detail in the preceding technique-specific chapters. Typically, special instructions might advise a simple increase in fluid intake to stop constipation after a barium procedure or may request the observation of a skin puncture site and regular monitoring of a patient's temperature, pulse and blood pressure by ward staff following an angiogram (see Chapter 2). Any specific aftercare will be explained to patients and anyone accompanying them to the imaging department both verbally and in writing. Following more complex or invasive procedures, further leaflets will be given out after the examination explaining what has happened and what the patient can expect over the next few days. These leaflets will also include a contact telephone number in case people become unduly worried or experience unexpected complications.

Getting the examination results

Arguably, the most important aspect of any imaging investigation is the result – by definition, the result of a justified imaging investigation must have some influence on clinical management. Not surprisingly then, people will be anxious to find out the result of their imaging examination and they will also want to know when this will happen. There is usually a time interval between having an imaging examination and getting the result because the person performing the examination is often not the person responsible for interpreting the imaging appearances (see Chapter 8). The time between having any diagnostic investigation or therapeutic procedure and getting the result is often very stressful, with many people expecting the worst and some convinced they have a serious illness or condition that cannot be alleviated. Imaging department staff know the importance of the investigation result and many Schemes of Work are in place to ensure imaging reports are generated and communicated to health care staff colleagues, to be passed on to patients, in a timely manner.

In a trauma situation and for hospital in-patients (namely those who have had accidents and/or who are already in hospital) the actual images might be sent with patients to be evaluated by a doctor or specially trained specialist nurse practitioner in the Accident and Emergency department or on the ward. Immediate decisions can then be made as to discharging people home or instigating appropriate treatment. The imaging department might operate a red-dot system (see Chapter 8), or alternatively a 'hot reporting' system where a radiologist or suitably trained radiographer will give an immediate examination report which is sent to the Accident and Emergency department or ward at the same time as the patient is returned.

Case study

Corrine was waiting to see Miss Wilson, the breast surgeon, after having her **mammogram** and breast ultrasound examinations. She had already been waiting 20 minutes and thought she would ask the nurse how much longer she would have to wait. Sue, the breast care nurse, apologised for the wait but explained that Dr Stephens had just looked at the images and was discussing the results with Miss Wilson. Ten minutes later, Miss Wilson explained to Corrine that Dr Stephens wanted to do a **biopsy** – to get a small sample of the lump that Corrine could feel in her breast. Corrine was relieved to know that this could be done today and would only take about 20 minutes, although she would have to wait another half an hour. Miss Wilson explained that the biopsy results would be available a few days later and that Corrine would be given an appointment before she left today.

Professional note

A **one-stop clinic** incorporates a 'hot reporting' system whereby several specialist practitioners undertake a range of diagnostic procedures and make the results available during a single clinic visit. Although such clinics typically mean patients spend quite a long time at the hospital, it is hoped that any inconvenience is offset by reducing the stress of waiting for results and further tests.

For most imaging examinations an immediate management decision is not required and the images are reviewed a short time after the examination once the imaged person has left the department. This is known as 'cold reporting'; it allows time to review the images in detail and consult with specialist colleagues or the medical literature if necessary. Although the time frames within which 'cold reports' are available will vary, all imaging departments do try to minimise these – electronic systems such as a PACS and voice recognition software help to reduce report turn-around times.

Confidentiality

Once a person has left the department and their results have been dispatched, imaging department staff will retain responsibility for keeping imaging records (images and reports) safe and secure. In accordance with the Data Protection Act 1998 records must be kept confidential and, in accordance with IR(ME)R 2000, records must be available at a later date to prevent the performance of unnecessary or repeat examinations. Typically, records are maintained electronically on password protected systems or are stored in locations with restricted access. Hospitals are required to appoint specific people, known as 'Caldicott guardians', to have responsibility for protecting the confidentiality of patient information and ensuring its legal and ethical use (DoH, 1999).

SUMMARY

A modern medical imaging department will be staffed by a wide range of highly trained and specialised health care professionals. It will also be equipped with a variety of complex technical equipment and will undertake a diverse series of routine and specialised techniques and procedures. It is not surprising that when people visit the department, either as members of the public or as health carers, they will sometimes find it a bewildering experience. Imaging department staff members are trained carers and will have had the experience of looking after people with a wide range of clinical conditions and from various social circumstances. The effectiveness of imaging examination procedures is improved when those attending for examinations, and those accompanying them as either social or professional supporters, are well informed and are encouraged to become fully involved in the care experience.

FURTHER READING

BMA (2006) *Consent and Capacity*. London: British Medical Association. Available at: **www.bma.org.uk/ap.nsf/Content/Hubethicsconsentand capacity**

DoH (2007) *Consent*. London: Department of Health. Available at: **www.dh.gov.uk/en/Policyandguidance/Healthandsocialcare topics/Consent/index.htm**

Ehrlich, R. A., McCloskey, E.D. and Daly, J.A. (2004) *Patient Care in Radiography* (6th Ed). London: Mosby

RCR (2005) *Standards for Patient Consent Particular to Radiology* (BFCR(05)8). London: Royal College of Radiologists

Glossary

acoustic boundary An interface between tissues that have different acoustic impedance values.

acoustic impedance A property of tissue density and compressibility that determines the speed at which sound travels through it.

acoustic shadow An area of reduced brightness in the ultrasound image behind strongly reflecting acoustic boundaries.

ALARP (As Low As Reasonably Practicable) – a philosophy of keeping potential for biological hazard to a minimum.

algorithm A rule for processing image data for storage or display – different algorithms can be used to 'sharpen' or 'soften' image appearances to optimise the display of specific anatomical features or disease processes.

allergy An adverse physiological reaction – may be mild (sneezing or itching) or severe (shortness of breath or heart attack).

aneurysm Abnormal widening of a blood vessel.

angina Chest pain caused by inadequate blood supply to the heart.

angiography Fluoroscopic examination of blood vessels after administration of contrast agent.

anode A positively charged component of the X-ray tube – attracts electrons given off by the tube filament (cathode) and converts the energy into X-rays.

antero-posterior (AP) projection Radiographic exposure made while the patient faces the X-ray tube: the X-rays pass through the body from anterior (front) to posterior (back).

artefact Anything that produces false readings in the image – may be caused by a computer/processing fault, patient's clothing, the presence of foreign bodies (including dentures and fillings).

artery A vessel taking blood from the heart to the rest of the body.

aseptic Sterile/free from infection.

aseptic conditions Using sterile equipment, wearing special clothing and surgical gloves.

aspiration Taking fluid out of a body cavity or cystic lesion.

atheroma Fatty deposits and calcium on the inner walls of blood vessels.

attenuation Dissipation/transfer of energy: in the body this is due to a combination of absorption, scattering and reflection. Although attenuation is what gives images their characteristic appearance, it is also the mechanism of biological damage.

authorised person Health care worker given official permission, on the basis of their professional training and qualifications, for restricted access to controlled areas.

automatic exposure control (AEC) An electronic device used to cut off radiation emission once an operator determined the threshold has been reached – used to optimise exposure settings and minimise patient dose.

barrier nursing Caring for patients using additional infection control precautions to reduce the risk of catching disease from a patient or to prevent transferring infection to an immunocompromised patient.

benign Localised and contained – the condition cannot spread to other sites in the body.

biopsy The removal of a small sample of tissue to examine under the microscope.

bypass surgery Creating an artificial channel to connect blood vessels (or bowel) above and below a diseased segment.

capillaries The smallest branches of blood vessels.

cassette A rigid box which houses the radiation detection device (photographic film or photostimulable plate).

catheter A flexible hollow tube inserted into a body cavity, hollow organ or blood vessel to introduce or drain fluid.

cathode The negatively charged component of the X-ray tube (filament) that generates electrons.

central venous catheter/line A soft tube inserted into a large vein, e.g. the superior vena cava, to monitor blood pressure and/or administer drugs.

chaperone A person present in the examination room who preserves the dignity of patients having intimate examinations or being examined by a health care worker of a different gender.

chronic obstructive pulmonary disease (COPD) Long-standing progressive lung disease.

claudication Pain in the legs caused by an inadequate blood supply.

clinical responsibility Has charge of a patient's care and management.

clotting factors Constituents of blood that are essential to stop bleeding.

colonoscopy A technique for looking inside the lumen of the colon (large bowel).

colour flow mapping Doppler ultrasound technique where information about moving structures is superimposed on the grey-scale image by colour coding the pixels corresponding to the moving structures.

Compton scattering A process by which X-ray photons change direction as a result of interaction with the nuclei of the body's atoms.

computed radiography A technique where a latent image is collected on a photostimulable plate and not on conventional photographic film.

computed tomography A radiation based imaging technique which collects and/or displays the body in cross-sectional slices.

conservative treatment A clinical management plan designed to avoid harm – usually avoids surgery and aggressive therapy using drugs with unpleasant side effects.

continuous spectrum Containing a variety of wavelengths.

contraindications Pre-existing conditions that make people more likely to have a bad reaction or complication to a procedure.

contrast agents Substances introduced into the body to alter its imaging characteristics.

contrast enhancement A technique for improving density differences between anatomical structures in an image by introducing either natural or artificial substances.

contrast resolution The ability to detect/display similar structures in the body at different greyscale levels in the image.

controlled area A space around a potentially hazardous substance/piece of equipment where access is restricted.

control room Where the CT and MRI scanner operator console is located – imaging staff remain here while the scan is in process to set and adjust the exposure parameters and ensure they are protected from any hazardous biological effects.

co-registration Simultaneous overlaid display of images acquired using two different techniques, e.g. PET-CT images.

coronal A longitudinal plane that divides the body into front and back sections.

coronary care A hospital ward specialising in looking after patients after heart attacks.

coupling gel An inert watery substance used between the ultrasound transducer and a person's skin to eliminate air and ensure good sound transmission in and out of the body.

creatinine A metabolic waste product – measured in blood or urine, to indicate renal function.

degenerative diseases Conditions associated with reduced function due to general 'wear and tear' as people get older.

delegate/delegation The legal process of transferring care from one health care professional to another.

detector A device used to capture image information (X-rays, gamma rays, sound waves, radiofrequency signals) coming through or from a patient during an imaging examination.

deterministic effects Where an early tissue reaction occurs, the severity of which is proportional to the exposure dose, the effect may be absent below a certain threshold level of exposure.

diabetes mellitus A disease of the pancreas resulting in insufficient secretion of insulin.

differential absorption Characteristic pattern of transmission, scattering and absorption of radiation by bodily tissues (according to their atomic number) that produces the greyscale 'shadow' image.

differential diagnoses A list of possible diseases that would fit a person's clinical signs and symptoms and image appearances.

digital detector A device that captures and stores image information in electronic (rather than photographic) format.

digital image matrix A two-dimensional electronic memory store consisting of rows and columns of pixels.

digital radiography A system utilising the electronic capture, storage and display of images.

direct digital Imaging equipment that converts X-ray photon energy directly into electrical charge for storage, processing and display.

Doppler effect A change in frequency of sound when there is relative movement between the source and the observer.

dose A quantity of radiation.

dosimetry The monitoring of occupational exposure to radiation.

double contrast A fluoroscopic examination using a combination of positive and negative contrast agents.

dual-phase An examination where two sets of images of the same area are obtained at two different physiological phases, e.g. to see arteries and veins after a contrast agent injection.

ectopic Located in the 'wrong' place – commonly used to refer to a pregnancy in the fallopian tube rather than the uterus.

effective dose A dose quantity that correlates with actual risk by taking into account the specific organs irradiated as well as the type of radiation.

electromagnetic induction The generation of an electric current by a changing magnetic field (and vice versa).

electron A negatively charged particle that orbits the nucleus of an atom.

electronic patient record An entry in a national computer database of all NHS records.

endogastric tube A soft tube introduced through the abdominal wall into a patient's stomach for feeding.

endometrium The lining of the uterus (womb) that is shed during menstruation.

endoscope A tubular device containing a fibre optic camera which can be inserted into the body.

endovascular device A medical device introduced through the skin into the lumen of a blood vessel.

end-stage renal failure Irreversible severe kidney damage that would normally result in death.

exit port A small window in the X-ray tube lead lining that allows X-rays to escape.

exposure A period of time over which X-rays are emitted during radiography.

exposure factors/parameters Operator controlled settings that determine the amount and quality of radiation used for imaging examinations.

fibroids Benign tumours in the wall of the uterus (womb) consisting of fatty and muscular tissue (leiomyomas).

field of view A cross-sectional area of tissue displayed in the image.

fistula An abnormal connection between two hollow channels in the body.

fluoroscopy A radiographic technique used to display moving structures in real-time.

fractures Broken bones.

gallstones Hard pebble-like collections of bile pigment, cholesterol and calcium salts that accumulate in the gallbladder or bile ducts – usually associated with inflammation and pain in the upper right quadrant of the abdomen.

gamma camera A radiation detection device used in nuclear medicine.

gamma rays Very short wavelength electromagnetic radiation given off by some radioactive materials – used to generate nuclear medicine images.

gantry The square 'doughnut' shaped stand that houses the X-ray tube and radiation detectors (CT) or magnets (MR) in a scanner.

geometric unsharpness The blurring of images caused by the mathematical relationships of the position, size of and/or relative distances between the radiation source, patient and detection device.

gestational age An estimate of the duration of a pregnancy calculated from either the date of a woman's last menstrual period or from ultrasound measurements of an embryo/fetus – the normal gestation of a human pregnancy is 40 weeks.

grey-scale The spectrum of monochrome shades between black and white used to represent anatomical structures in medical images.

gynaecology The area of medicine covering disorders of the female reproductive system.

haemostasis The stoppage of bleeding achieved naturally through blood vessel constriction and clotting physically by applying direct pressure, or surgically by cauterisation, stitching or pharmaceutical sealing.

half-life The time taken for the amount of radioactivity present in a given volume of radiopharmaceutical to reduce by 50 per cent.

hard copy Data/information stored and/or viewed on paper/photographic film.

hot spots Areas of increased density on radionuclide images representing anatomical areas of increased radiotracer uptake; may indicate fracture, inflammation or tumour.

Hounsfield unit (HU) The numeric value used in CT to describe attenuation properties of tissue.

hydrated Having enough fluid in the body to carry out normal functional processes.

image intensifier A component of fluoroscopy equipment which amplifies the light signal from the X-ray exposure to a level suitable for display on a TV monitor.

immunocompromised Having reduced resistance to infection.

indirect digital An imaging system that converts X-ray energy into light and then into an electrical charge for storage and display.

informed consent The permission given by a patient to carry out procedures after being given an understandable explanation of the proposed activity.

intensifying screens Thin sheets of plastic coated on one side with luminescent material that are attached to the insides of an X-ray cassette – intensifying screens emit light when irradiated and thus enhance the film blackening effect of X-ray photons.

intensive care The specialised treatment and monitoring of people who are critically ill or unstable, including the giving of support to maintain essential bodily functions.

internal fixation device Surgical plates and screws inserted to hold broken bones together.

international normalised ratio (INR) A measure of how long it takes a person's blood to clot compared to the normal average value.

inverse square law A physical rule describing the relationship between radiation intensity and the distance from its source – if staff working in radiation environments stand twice as far away from a radiation source they quarter their radiation dose.

ionising radiation High energy radiation that can knock electrons out of their atomic orbit.

IR(ME)R 2000 The main legislation governing the use of ionising radiation in medicine.

ischaemia Inadequate blood supply.

isocentre The point at which three separate dimensional planes converge.

isolation Total separation from surroundings.

justified/justify/justification The legal process of confirming that a medical imaging investigation request is appropriate.

kidney stones Hard pebble-like masses usually containing calcium that form in the kidney – often associated with inflammation and pain in the back and/or groin.

lateral projection A radiographic exposure made while the patient's side is nearest the X-ray tube – the X-rays pass through the body from left to right (or vice versa).

lesion A focal area of abnormal tissue – may be benign or malignant.

light beam diaphragm X-ray tube attachment, containing lead-lined shutters and a visible light source aligned with the X-ray beam, that shows the location of the X-ray beam on the surface of a patient's body and helps the radiographer control the position and area of irradiation.

line spectra Photons of a discrete energy produced when electrons interact with the orbiting electrons of the tungsten target atoms.

lumen The innermost channel of a hollow tube such as the bowel or a blood vessel.

magnetic moment A measure of the effective strength of a magnetic source.

magnetic resonance imaging (MRI) A non-radiation based imaging technique that uses magnetic fields to image hydrogen atoms in the body.

malignancy A condition that is capable of breaching local tissue boundaries and spreading to other areas of the body.

mammogram A radiographic examination of the breasts – utilises specialist equipment optimised to give high spatial and contrast resolution.

matrix An array of rows and columns of pixels or voxels used to store or display digital images – a matrix with a large number of elements can display information at high resolution.

metabolism/metabolic The biological rate of chemical and physical function and growth.

metastasis/metastases/metastatic Secondary malignant tumours occurring due to the spread of a primary tumour.

morbidity The adverse events/complications associated with a condition/procedure.

multidisciplinary team A group of health care workers from different professional backgrounds working together closely to care for patients with a particular condition.

multiplanar reformatting (MPR) The digital manipulation of stored image data to allow viewing in different planes without having to re-position and expose the patient again.

multiple myeloma A malignant disease of bone marrow/plasma cells.

myocardial infarction A heart attack – the heart muscle dies due to insufficient oxygenated blood supply.

naso-gastric tube A soft tube introduced into a patient's stomach via their nose – can be used for feeding, or draining the stomach contents.

noise Random electronic (or other) interference that degrades image quality.

nuchal thickness A measurement made at the back of an unborn baby's neck to assess the risk of Down's syndrome.

occult A condition that has no outward signs and symptoms.

one-stop clinic Out-patient services where a patient gets all the necessary tests, investigations and results in a single visit.

PACS Patient Archiving and Communication System – a centralised electronic facility for storing, retrieving, distributing and displaying images.

parameter The technical functions that radiographers set and/or alter during imaging examinations to control exposure conditions and optimise image quality.

pathological Relating to a diseased state.

perforation An abnormal hole in the wall of a hollow organ or channel.

perfusion The passage of fluid (usually blood) through tissues.

peripheral vascular disease A disease of blood vessels other than those supplying the heart and brain; fatty deposits on the inner walls of arteries narrow the lumen and restrict blood supply.

photodiode A device that converts light into either current or voltage.

photoelectric absorption A process where all the energy of an X-ray photon is transferred to an atom within the body – as all the energy is 'absorbed' by the patient none emerges to hit the image detector.

photomultiplier tube A device for converting small amounts of photon (light) energy into usable electric current.

photon The smallest unit of electromagnetic radiation.

photostimulable image plate A thin phosphor coated plastic sheet used in the cassette of a computed radiography system that absorbs X-ray photons during exposure, stores the latent image as electric charges and later releases the energy when stimulated with a scanning laser beam.

physiology Pertaining to functions of the body and its parts.

piezoelectric The process of converting electrical energy to mechanical energy (and vice versa).

pixel One of the picture elements making up a digital image.

pneumonia An infection of lung tissue which causes the air sacs to fill with pus.

pneumothorax Air in the pleural space – compresses and collapses the lung.

polyp A small overgrowth of tissue – usually arising from the lining of a hollow organ and protruding into its cavity.

postero-anterior (PA) projection A radiographic exposure made while the patient faces the detector – X-rays pass through the body from posterior (back) to anterior (front).

pre-op chest A radiograph of the chest performed prior to surgery.

primary An original (first) tumour.

proforma A standard outline (e.g. report form) prepared in advance – ensures consistency of style, enables rapid completion and avoids unnecessary repetition of set phrases.

prognosis The assessment of the future course and outcome of a condition/disease.

projection A radiographic positioning and exposure technique.

prosthesis An artificial body part, e.g. a metal joint replacement, a silicone breast implant.

protocol A set of guidelines customised for a specific examination or disease process to ensure consistency of the examination technique/clinical practice.

proton A positively charged subatomic particle in the nucleus of an atom.

pulse sequence A combination of scanning parameters/exposure conditions used in magnetic resonance imaging.

radiation dose A measure of radiation energy used to quantify associated risk.

radioactive Materials containing disintegrating atomic nuclei.

radioactive decay The emission of subatomic particles/electromagnetic radiation from a disintegrating atom.

radiographer A non-medical health care professional trained and registered to operate medical imaging equipment.

radiographic contrast Differences in density displayed in the radiographic image as a result of the different attenuating properties of structures in the body.

radiographic density Grey-scale values on a conventional radiographic image.

radiologist A doctor specialising in medical imaging techniques and interpretation.

radionuclide The radioactive version of a chemical element.

radio-opaque Absorbs radiation to prevent it reaching a detector.

radiopharmaceutical A combined radionuclide and pharmaceutical preparation administered to patients for scintigraphy examinations.

radiosensitivity A measure of the susceptibility of tissue to damage from radiation exposure.

radiotherapy A medical specialism using radiation to treat (destroy) tumours.

radiotracer A combined radionuclide/pharmaceutical preparation used in nuclear medicine examinations that is taken up or accumulates in a particular area of the body.

'red dot' system A system of annotating images with an identifying mark to show that an abnormality may have been demonstrated.

referred/referral The legal process of delegating medical care from one doctor to another – the process by which medical imaging investigation requests are made.

replication The process of DNA duplication during cell division.

report The permanent legal record of the imaging examination.

request The legal referral of a patient for a medical imaging investigation/procedure.

respiratory tract The body system responsible for breathing – nose/mouth, pharynx, trachea and lungs.

role extension Professional development to undertake responsibilities and practices not covered in initial training.

Royal College of Radiologists (RCR) The professional body representing doctors who have specialised in medical imaging.

safety screening The process of checking that patients and visitors entering the MRI unit are not at increased risk of adverse effects.

sagittal The longitudinal plane that divides the body into right and left sections.

scanogram An initial CT image of a large area of the body used to plan the start and finish levels of the actual examination.

scattered radiation Radiation that has been changed in direction, quantity and/or quality (energy level).

Scheme of Work A standardised and agreed system of professional practice.

screening The systematic investigation of people without signs and symptoms to detect early and/or occult (hidden) disease.

sensitivity The extent to which a test is positive when an abnormality is truly present.

sinus An abnormal channel or false track into the body.

skeleton The bony framework which supports the body and protects the soft tissue organs.

soft copy Data stored electronically and viewed on a TV monitor.

space occupying lesion A tumour that displaces surrounding tissue as it grows and expands.

spatial resolution The ability to display fine anatomical detail by showing small closely spaced structures as being separate.

specificity The extent to which a test is negative when no abnormality is present.

Spectral Doppler The Doppler ultrasound technique where information about moving structures is shown in graphical format.

stable Unchanging – a patient whose condition is not getting better or worse.

stage/staging The process of determining the full extent or spread of a disease and classifying it according to a recognised scale.

stenosis The narrowing of a channel, e.g. blood vessel or bowel.

stent An artificial flexible tubular structure inserted into the lumen of a hollow organ, vessel or duct to keep blood or other fluid flowing.

stochastic effects A random effect in which the severity of radiation hazard is independent of the magnitude of the exposure dose but the probability of the effect is proportional to the exposure dose.

stroke A medical condition where part of the brain dies – usually due to a loss of blood supply.

systemic circulation The network of blood vessels supplying and draining the human body (the pulmonary circulation circulates blood between the heart and the lungs for oxygen/carbon dioxide exchange).

target The component of an X-ray tube bombarded with electrons to produce X-rays.

telemedicine The use of secure internet connections to send and receive images between hospitals/doctors.

Tesla A unit of magnetic field strength.

thrombolytic Possessing the ability to dissolve blood clots.

time-activity curve A graph showing how activity (of a radionuclide or radiographic/sonographic contrast agent) changes over time.

tissue reactions Adverse effects of radiation exposure that are apparent soon after exposure (see deterministic effects).

transabdominal An ultrasound examination performed through the anterior abdominal wall.

transducer A commonly used term for the handheld device containing piezoelectric material that is placed in contact with a patient to generate sound pulses and detect echo signals during ultrasound examinations.

transvaginal An ultrasound examination performed by placing a long narrow transducer into a woman's vagina.

ultrasound A medical imaging technique using high frequency (MegaHertz range) sound waves.

uptake The physiological process whereby a radiopharmaceutical is extracted from the blood, or accumulates, in an organ/area of the body.

virtual surgery The electronic technique of 'dissolving' tissue (on CT images) to display structures that would otherwise only be seen during an operation.

voxel A discrete element of the digital memory store representing a volume of tissue.

windowing A computer process for altering the range of values of stored data that is viewed in the displayed image – in CT, for example, this allows viewing of the lungs and soft tissues and the bony thorax without the need for irradiating the patient twice.

X-ray exposures Controlled events where limited amounts of X-radiation are used to generate images of the body.

X-rays Short wavelength electromagnetic radiation used to generate radiography, fluoroscopy and computed tomography images.

X-ray tube An evacuated glass tube in which electrons are accelerated at high speed towards a tungsten target to generate X-rays.

References

ARSAC (2006) *Notes for Guidance on the Clinical Administration of Radiopharmaceuticals and Use of Sealed Radioactive Sources* (March). Didcot, Oxon: Administration of Radioactive Substances Advisory Committee, Health Protection Agency. Available online at: **www.arsac.org.uk/notes_for_guidence/index.htm** (7 March 2008)

Benya, E.C., Lim-Dunham, J.E., Landrum, O. and Statter, M. (2000) 'Abdominal sonography in examination of children with blunt abdominal trauma'. *American Journal of Roentgenology*, 174: 1613–1616

Bolus, N.E. (2001) 'Basic review of radiation biology and terminology'. *Journal of Nuclear Medicine Technology*, 29(2): 67–73. Available online at: **http://tech.snmjournals.org/cgi/reprint/29/2/67.pdf** (27 March 2008)

Brenner, D.J., Doll, R., Goodhead, D.T., Halla, E.J., Lande, C.E., Little, J.B., Lubin, J.H., Preston, D.L., Preston, R.J., Puskin, J.S., Ron, E., Sachs, R.K., Samet, J.M., Setlow, R.B. and Zaider, M. (2003) 'Cancer risks attributable to low doses of ionizing radiation: Assessing what we really know'. *Proceedings of the National Academy of Sciences*, 100(24): 13761–13766. Available online at: **www.pnas.org/cgi/reprint/223559 2100v1** (27 March 2008)

Bronshtein, M., Nussem, D. and Blumenfeld, Z. (1996) 'Transvaginal ultrasound may cause latex anaphylaxis'. *Ultrasound in Obstetrics and Gynecology*, 7(5): 379–380

Caseiro-Alves, F., Brito, J., Araujo, A.E., Belo-Soares, P., Rodrigues, H., Cipriano, A., Sousa, D. and Mathieu, D. (2007) 'Liver haemangioma: common and uncommon findings and how to improve the differential diagnosis'. *European Radiology*, 17(6): 1544–1554

Chapman, S. and Nakielny, R. (2001) *A Guide to Radiological Procedures* (4th Ed). Edinburgh: Saunders

Chudleigh, T. and Thilaganathan, B. (2004) *Obstetric Ultrasound: How, Why & When?* (3rd Ed). Edinburgh: Elsevier Churchill Livingstone

Data Protection Act (1999) (c.29) London: HMSO

DEFRA (2008) *The Justification of Practices Involving Ionising Radiation Regulations 2004 SI2004 Nov. 1769. - Guidance on their Application and Administration* v. May 2008 (online). London: DEFRA (Radioactive Substances Division). Available at: **www.defra.gov.uk/environment/radioactivity/government/legislation/pdf/regulations guidelines.pdf** (4 August 2008)

Dendy, P.P. and Heaton, B. (1999) *Physics for Diagnostic Radiology* (2nd Ed). Bristol: Institute of Physics Publishing

DoH (1999) *Caldicott Guardians in the NHS* (HSC1999/012). London: Department of Health

DoH (2000) *The NHS Plan: A Plan for Investment A Plan for Reform* (CM48C8-I, July). London: Department of Health

DoH (2001) *Reference Guide to Consent for Examination or Treatment* (23617). London: Department of Health. Available at: **www.dh.gov.uk/en/Publicationsandstatistics/Publications/PublicationsPolicyAndGuidance/DH_4006757** (4 April 2008)

DoH (2005) (online) *NHS Connecting for Health*. Available at **www.connectingfor health.nhs.uk** (21 December 2007)

Dowsett, D.J., Kenny, P.A. and Johnston, R.E. (2006) *The Physics of Diagnostic Imaging* (2nd Ed). London: Hodder Arnold

EFSUMB (2006) *Clinical Safety Statement for Diagnostic Ultrasound* (rev. 4), London: European Federation of Societies for Ultrasound in Medicine and Biology

Farr, R.F. and Allisy-Roberts, P.J. (1998) *Physics for Medical Imaging*. Edinburgh: WB Saunders, Harcourt

Fry, A., Meagher, S. and Vollenhoven, B. (1999) 'A case of anaphylactic reaction caused by exposure to a latex probe cover in transvaginal ultrasound scanning'. *Ultrasound in Obstetrics and Gynecology*, 13(5): 373.

Garcia, J., Bricker, L., Henderson, J., Martin, M-A., Mugford, M., Nielson, J. and Roberts, T. (2002) 'Women's views of pregnancy ultrasound: a systematic review'. *Birth*, 29 (4): 225–250

GMC (1998) *Seeking Patients' Consent: The Ethical Considerations*. London: General Medical Council. Available at **www.gmc-uk.org/guidance/current/library/consent. asp#33** (4 April 2008)

GMC (2006) *Good Medical Practice*. London: General Medical Council

Graham, D.T. and Cloke, P. (2003) *Principles of Radiological Physics* (3rd Ed). London: Elsevier Churchill Livingstone

Hart, D., Jones, D.G. and Wall, B.F. (1994) *Estimation of Effective Doses in Diagnostic Radiology from Entrance Surface Dose and Dose-Area Product Measurements*. (NRPB-R262). Chilton: National Radiological Protection Board

Health Committee (2007) *Sixth Report: The Electronic Patient Record* (HC 422-I). London: Health Committee

HPA (2001) *X-rays: How Safe Are They?* (online). Didcot, Oxon: National Radiological Protection Board (now Health Protection Agency – Radiation Protection Division). Available at: **www.hpa.org.uk/radiation/default.htm** (29 February 2008)

HSE (1999) *Ionising Radiations Regulations 1999 Approved Code of Practice and Guidance* (L 121). London: HSE Books

ICRP (2007) *Recommendations of the International Commission on Radiological Protection*. (ICRP Publication 103). Stockholm: ICRP

IR(ME)R (2000) *Ionising Radiations (Medical Exposure) Regulations (2000)* (SI 1059) (online). London: The Stationery Office. Available at: **www.opsi.gov.uk/si/si2000/ 20001059.htm** (27 March 2008)

IRR (1999) *The Ionising Radiations Regulations 1999* (SI.3232). London: The Stationery Office. Available online at: **www.legislation.gov.uk/si/si1999/19993232.htm** (27 March 2008)

Justification of Practices Involving Ionising Radiation Regulations SI2004. No. 1769. London: The Stationery Office. Available online at: **www.opsi.gov.uk/si/si2004/20041769. htm** (27 March 2008)

Kalender, W.A., Seissler, W., Klotz, E. and Vock, P. (1990) 'Spiral volumetric CT with single-breathhold technique, continuous transport, and continuous scanner rotation'. *Radiology* 176(1): 181–183

Kessel, D. and Robertson, I. (2005) *Interventional Radiology: A Survival Guide* (2nd Ed). Edinburgh: Elsevier, Churchill Livingstone

MARS (1978) *The Medicines (Administration of Radioactive Substances) Regulations 1978 (SI 1978 1006)*. London: HMSO

Medicines & Healthcare Products Regulatory Agency (MHRA) (2007) *Device Bulletin – Safety Guidelines for Magnetic Resonance Imaging Equipment in Clinical Use: (DB2007(03))*. London: Department of Health

Meinhold, C.B. and Taschner, J.C. (1995) 'A brief history of radiation (in Radiation and Risk – A hard look at the data.)'. *Los Alamos Science*, 23: 16. Available online at: **www.fas.org/sgp/othergov/doe/lanl/00326630.pdf** (27 March 2008)

Moir, D. (2005) *Assessment and Management of Risks from Radiological Hazards*. Ontario: Health Canada. Available at: **www.who.int/peh-emf/meetings/archive/moir_ottawa july05.pdf** (29 February 2008)

Mortazavi, M.J. (no date) *An Introduction to Radiation Hormesis*. Available online at: **www.angelfire.com/mo/radioadaptive/inthorm.html** (27 March 2008.)

NICE (2001) *Management of Stroke* (under review, due to be released 2008). London: National Institute for Clinical Excellence

NICE (2003a) *Triage, Assessment, Investigation and Early Management of Head Injuries in Infants, Children and Adults*. (Clinical Guideline 4: June). London: National Institute for Clinical Excellence

NICE (2003b) *Antenatal Care: Routine Care for the Healthy Pregnant Woman*. (Clinical Guideline 6). London: National Institute for Clinical Excellence

NICE (2005) *Lung Cancer, Diagnosis and Treatment* (Clinical Guideline 24: February). London: National Institute for Clinical Excellence

NICE (2007) *Head Injury: Triage, Assessment, Investigation and Early Management of Head Injury in Infants, Children and Adults* (Clinical Guideline 56: partial update of Clinical Guideline 4: September) London: National Institute for Clinical Excellence

NRPB (1990) *National Protocol for Patient Dose Measurements in Diagnostic Radiology* NRPB 1(3): Dosimetry Working Party of the Institute of Physical Sciences in Medicine). Chilton, Oxon: Health Protection Agency Centre for Radiation, Chemical and Environmental Hazards. Available online at: **www.hpa.org.uk/radiation/publications/misc_publications/national_protocol.htm** (27 March 2008)

Olson, J.S. (2002) *Bathsheba's Breast: Women, Cancer and History*. Baltimore: Johns Hopkins University Press

ONS (2005) 'Deaths by age, sex and underlying cause, 2004 registrations'. *Health Statistics Quarterly*, 26. Available at: **www.statistics.gov.uk/STATBASE/Expodata/Spreadsheets/D8986.xls** (12 June 2008).

ONS (2007) *Population Estimates*. Available at: **www.statistics.gov.uk/cci/nugget.asp?id=6** (12 June 2008).

RCN (2007) *Clinical Imaging Requests from Non-Medically Qualified Professionals*. London: Royal College of Nursing

RCP (2004) *National Clinical Guidelines for Stroke 2004*. London: Royal College of Physicians

RCR (1998) *Intimate Examinations* (BFCR(98)5). London: Royal College of Radiologists

RCR (1999) *Good Practice for Clinical Radiologists* (BFCR(99)11). London: Royal College of Radiologists

RCR (2005) *Ultrasound Training Recommendations for Medical and Surgical Specialties* (BFCR(05)2). London: Royal College of Radiologists

RCR (2006) *Recommendations for Cross-Sectional Imaging in Cancer Management*. (BFCR(06)1). London: Royal College of Radiologists

RCR (2007) *Making Best Use of Clinical Radiology Services* (MBUR6) (BFCR(07)10). London: Royal College of Radiologists

RCR/SoR (2007) *Team Working Within Clinical Imaging: A Contemporary View of Skills Mix* (BFCR(07)1). London: Royal College of Radiologists, Society of Radiographers

Shope, T.B. (1995) 'Radiation-induced skin injuries from fluoroscopy'. *Radiology*, 197(P) S449. Available online at: **www.fda.gov/cdrh/rsnaii.html** (27 March 2008)

SoR (2007) *Consent to Imaging and Radiotherapy Treatment Examinations: An Ethical Perspective and Good Practice Guide for the Radiography Workforce*. London: Society of Radiographers

Szczepura, A. and Clark, M.D. (2000) 'Creating a strategic management plan for magnetic resonance imaging (MRI) Provision'. *Health Policy*, 53: 91–104 (0168-8510)

Thompson, C. and Wakeling, J. (2003) *AS-Level Physics: The Revision Guide*. Kirkby-in-Furness: Coordination Group

Watson, S.J., Jones, A.L., Oatway, W.B. and Hughes, J.S. (2005) *Ionising Radiation Exposure of the UK Population: 2005 Review*. Didcot: Health Protection Agency

Westbrook, C., Kaut, C.K. and Talbot, J. (2005) *MRI in Practice* (3rd Ed). Oxford: Blackwell

Whittle, M.J., Chitty, L.S., Neilson, J.P. *et al.* (2000) *Ultrasound Screening*. London: RCOG. Available online at **www.rcog.org.uk/print.asp?PageID=439&Type=main** (7 March 2005)

Index

Note: the letter 'f' after a page number refers to a figure; the letter 't' refers to a table.

flat panel LCD monitors 11
fluid, free 16, 72, 109, 110f, 119,
  143
fluid-filled structures 101
fluid intake *see* hydration
Fluorine-18 (F18) 94
fluorodeoxyglucose (FDG) 94
fluoroscopy
  biological hazard 163
  case studies 32, 35–7, 39, 45–6
  clinical applications
    barium enema 33–7, 33f, 34f,
      35f
    interventional radiography
      37–46, 38t, 39f, 40–1f, 42–
      3f, 54, 166, 175–6
    pancreas examinations 109
  contrast agents
    choice, administration and
      elimination 27, 29f, 30
    and interventional
      radiography 39, 44, 45
    principles of use 24–6, 25f
    side effects 30–2, 31t
    types 26, 27f, 28f, 29t
  definition 22
  equipment 22–4, 23f
  radiation protection for staff 24,
    54–5
food 24, 63
  see also diet restrictions; fasting
foreign bodies 19–20, 19f, 134t,
  150
  see also artefacts; implants;
    pacemakers; prostheses
fractures
  bone scintigraphy 86, 94
  computed tomography (CT) 72
  dental radiography 19
  magnetic resonance imaging
    (MRI) 72, 143
  orthopaedic radiography 16,
    166
free fluid 16, 72, 109, 110f, 119,
  143

frequency
  in ultrasound 102, 103, 105
friends *see* accompanying
  supporters; person/family-
  centred care; radiological
  protection for general public
Fry, A. 111

gadolinium 32, 135–6, 137–9f,
  139, 140–1f, 145
gall bladder 18, 109
gallstones 18, 109
gamma camera
  and radionuclide imaging/
    scintigraphy 75, 76f, 79–81,
    85, 85f, 86f, 89
  and SPECT (single photon
    emission computed
    tomography) 90, 93
gamma rays 1, 3t, 75, 78, 79, 84,
  94
gantry 48–9, 49f, 56, 65, 130
Garcia, J. 112
gas *see* air
gastrointestinal tract
  computed tomography (CT) 65
  contrast agents in fluoroscopy
    24, 25, 29t, 30
  fluoroscopic guided intervention
    38t
  general radiography 19f
  magnetic resonance imaging
    (MRI) 145, 148, 148f
Gauss 149
general public *see* accompanying
  supporters; person/family-
  centred care; radiological
  protection for general public
general radiography
  case studies 5, 7, 13
  clinical uses 14–19, 15f, 14, 17f,
    18f, 19f, 20f, 72, 109, 149,
    166, 167
  contrast agents 7, 168
  patients – preparation and

Index

235

optimisation 172–3
radionuclide imaging/
    scintigraphy 75, 81, 81f
ultrasound 100
virtual surgery 72–3
visible light 3t
visitors *see* accompanying
    supporters; person/family-
    centred care; radiological
    protection for general public
voxels 50

water 50, 53f, 63, 64t, 65f, 124,
    135
see also hydration; urine
water-soluble iodine based contrast
    agents
    contraindications 30–1, 188–9
    computed tomography (CT)
        64t, 65
    fluoroscopy 25f, 29t, 30–1, 32,
        39, 45
    and radionuclide imaging/
        scintigraphy 84
Watson, S.J. 14
wavelength, electromagnet
    radiation 1, 3t

Westbrook, C. 151
wheelchairs 150, 182
Whittle, M.J. 113
windowing, in CT 61

X plane in MRI 127f, 132
X-ray tube
    computed tomography (CT)
        48–9, 49f, 56, 56f, 65
    fluoroscopy 23, 23f
    general radiography 2–4, 4f, 8f
X-ray tube current (mAs) 60
X-rays
    defined 1, 3t
    discovery 1, 153
    effect on the body 5–7, 6f, 7f
    production 1–4, 3t, 4f
X-ray viewing box 11, 11f, 172–3

Y plane in MRI 127f, 132
young people 144
    see also babies; children; unborn
        babies

Z plane in MRI 127f, 132